Semiconductor Quantum Dots and Rods for In Vivo Imaging and Cancer Phototherapy

Semiconductor Quantum Dots and Rods for In Vivo Imaging and Cancer Phototherapy

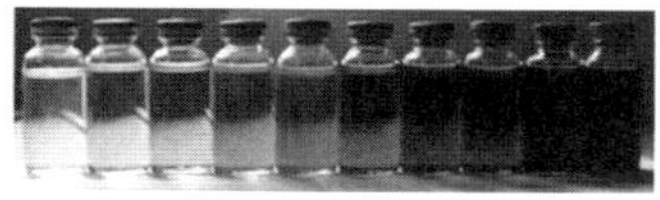

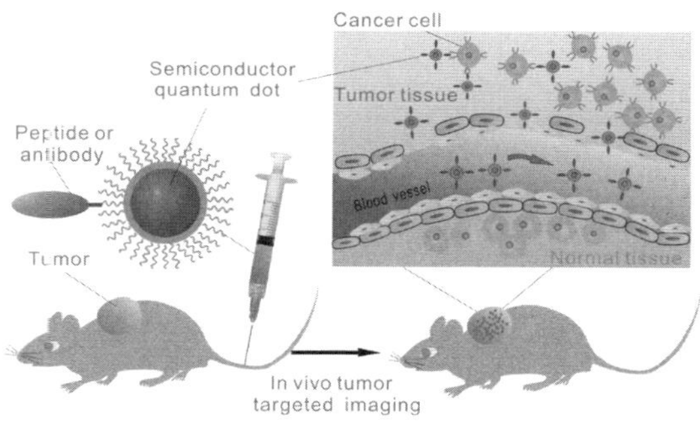

Maoquan Chu
Tongji University, China

World Scientific

NEW JERSEY · LONDON · SINGAPORE · BEIJING · SHANGHAI · HONG KONG · TAIPEI · CHENNAI · TOKYO

Published by

World Scientific Publishing Co. Pte. Ltd.
5 Toh Tuck Link, Singapore 596224
USA office: 27 Warren Street, Suite 401-402, Hackensack, NJ 07601
UK office: 57 Shelton Street, Covent Garden, London WC2H 9HE

Library of Congress Cataloging-in-Publication Data
Names: Chu, Maoquan, author.
Title: Semiconductor quantum dots and rods for in vivo imaging and cancer phototherapy / Maoquan Chu (Tongji University, China).
Description: New Jersey : World Scientific, 2016. | Includes bibliographical references.
Identifiers: LCCN 2016014417 | ISBN 9789813142886 (hc : alk. paper)
Subjects: | MESH: Neoplasms--therapy | Phototherapy--methods | Quantum Dots | Diagnostic Imaging--methods | Nanomedicine--methods
Classification: LCC RC270.3.D53 | NLM QZ 266 | DDC 616.99/40754--dc23
LC record available at https://lccn.loc.gov/2016014417

British Library Cataloguing-in-Publication Data
A catalogue record for this book is available from the British Library.

Desk Editors: Dr. Sree Meenakshi Sajani/Catherine Yeo

Typeset by Stallion Press
Email: enquiries@stallionpress.com

Printed in Singapore

Contents

Preface		vii
About the Author		xi
Chapter 1	Semiconductor Quantum Dots for Sentinel Lymph Node Mapping through *In Vivo* Fluorescent Imaging	1
Chapter 2	Semiconductor Quantum Dots for *In Vivo* Tumor-targeted Imaging	27
Chapter 3	Self-Illuminating Quantum Dots for *In Vivo* Imaging	49
Chapter 4	Semiconductor Quantum Rods with Bright Fluorescence and Slow Bleaching Kinetics for Cell Labeling and *In Vivo* Imaging	67
Chapter 5	Semiconductor Quantum Dots for Photodynamic Cancer Therapy	91
Chapter 6	Semiconductor Quantum Dots for Photothermal Cancer Therapy	111

Chapter 7 Semiconductor Quantum Dot-tagged Graphene Nanosheets for Bioimaging and Cancer Dual Modal Therapy 141

Chapter 8 Magnetic Quantum Dot Hybrid Nanocomposites for Multimodal Cancer Imaging and Therapy 157

Preface

Thousands of new cancer cases and deaths from cancer are recorded in the current world. Cancer might become the leading cause of death in the future. Many cases of cancer are diagnosed at an advanced incurable stage, and these patient lives are therefore hard to be saved. Early diagnosis and treatment are very important for declining the rate of death. In the past decades, novel techniques involved cancer diagnosis and therapy emerged in an endless stream. Nanotechnology may be one of the most attractive novel techniques in cancer research field. The applications of nanotechnologies to biology and medicine that involve cancer diagnosis and treatment is named as nanobiomedicine. Nanoparticles with only 1–100 nm in size usually have unique physical and/or chemical properties, which have attracted great attention in the research of cancer diagnosis and therapy. Preparation and biomedical applications of the nanoparticles are key contents in nanobiomedicine. Up to now, semiconductor nanocrystals including quantum dots (QDs) and quantum rods (QRs), magnetic nanoparticles, gold nanoparticles with specific morphologies, graphene nanosheets, polymer nanospheres, dendrimer, and micelle, etc., have been intensively investigated for drug delivery, biomedical imaging and tumor target therapy, which have shown many advantages over the traditional techniques.

Long-term tracing of the distribution and clearance of biomolecules and drugs in cells or in animal body or observing the interaction between the biomolecules or biomolecules and cells, or tracing cells migrating in living tissues are very important techniques in biomedical research field including cancer diagnosis and therapy. Among the nanoparticles as mentioned above, semiconductor QDs and QRs have unique and fascinating optical and electrical properties, which are excellent reagents for biolabeling and target tracing through fluorescent imaging.

Semiconductor QDs are inorganic nanocompounds composed of groups II(B)–VI(A) or III(A)–V(A) or IV(A)–VI(A) or II(B)–VI(A) or I(B)–VI(A) or I(B)–III(A)–VI(A) elements containing roughly 200–10,000 atoms. The sizes of these nanocrystals are only 1–10 nm, which are close to or smaller than the dimensions of exciton Bohr radius. QDs exhibit strong quantum size effect, which provides size-dependent fluorescent emission bands. Therefore, multicolored QDs with narrow emission peaks can be conveniently synthesized by controlling the QD size. Since the QDs have broad and continuous absorption spectra from ultraviolet (UV) to near-infrared (NIR), these multicolored QDs can be synchronously excited by a single light. This is a benefit for multiplexed imaging. Importantly, QD fluorescence is exceptionally bright and stable, which makes them good candidates for monitoring the long-term interactions of biomolecules in cells or monitoring other long-term biological processes including *in vivo* tumor targeting and imaging. These optical properties of the QDs are greatly superior to those of the conventional organic dyes.

In 1998, Nie's and Alivisatos's research groups synchronously reported that QDs could be used to label living cells. From then on, a great deal of work has been reported on the biomedical applications of the QDs all over the world. Beside the *in vitro* cancer cell labeling and imaging, *in vivo* sentinel lymph node (SLN) mapping and tumor target imaging are the very interesting research fields of the QDs. QDs are only several nanometers in diameter, they usually migrate into lymph vessels quickly after subcutaneous injection and then accumulate in SLNs for a long time via passive targeting. Therefore, NIR QDs are suitable for cancer SLN mapping through *in vivo* fluorescent imaging. Since NIR fluorescence in animal tissue can be detected without the incision of skin and muscle, SLN containing NIR QDs can be seen in real time, which would eliminate or reduce the need for surgical management. QDs can also passive target to solid tumor in animal body due to the enhanced permeability and retention (EPR) effect of tumor tissue. The *in vivo* tumor target efficiency of the QDs would be significantly improved by conjugation of antibody or peptide or other biorecognition molecules. This technique can be used for detecting where the solid tumor is located in body, which has potential for cancer diagnosis.

To decrease the interference of strong background autofluorescence and improve the tissue depth of detection, self-illuminating QDs based on bioluminescence resonance energy transfer (BRET) technique have been developed in recent years. Since no external excitation is required, *in vivo* bioluminescence imaging using the QD-BRET system have no background autofluorescence and may be applied for detecting the tissue at a depth of more than 2 cm beneath skin. Compared with the fluorescent imaging using QDs, however, the bioluminescence imaging using the QD-BRET system is not suitable for long-term detection since the amount of luciferase on the QD surface and substrate around the QD-luciferase system, as well as the bioactivity of the luciferase all decline with time.

QDs upon laser irradiation generate cytotoxic reactive oxygen species (ROS) such as singlet oxygen ($^1O_2$). Therefore, QDs especially the NIR QDs may be acted as photosensitizers for photodynamic therapy (PDT) of cancer in deep tissue. Unlike other molecular photosensitizers, QDs also release heavy metal ions into cancer cells after irradiation, which will further kill cancer cells. Importantly, QDs can convert laser light into heat energy, which has potential for cancer photothermal therapy (PTT). Therefore, NIR QDs upon laser irradiation will exhibit multimodal therapy: PDT + PTT + toxicity of the heavy ions. Cancer cells will be high efficiently killed by the synergistic effect of these three stimulation therapy methods. Animal experiments showed that the mouse tumors injected with cadmium-containing QDs finally disappeared after NIR laser irradiation.

After the QDs are incorporated into other interesting nanoparticles such as gold shell, magnetic nanoparticles, graphene nanosheets, etc., the novel nanocomposites obtained will exhibit strong biomedical functions. For example, a nanosphere containing QDs and magnetic iron oxide nanoparticles can be used for fluorescence and nuclear magnetic resonance double imaging, drug delivery, cancer PDT and PTT, and destroying cancer cells through magnetomechanical force or magnetic switch. For another example, the QD-graphene nanosheet hybrid nanocomposites can not only be used for fluorescent imaging, loading drugs, cancer PDT and PTT, but can also significantly reduce the QD toxicity.

Semiconductor QRs also have the interesting optical properties such as size-tunable emission wavelength, high quantum yield and strong resistance to photobleaching. Therefore, QRs also can be used for *in vitro* biolabeling, SLN mapping, *in vivo* tumor targeting imaging, as well as cancer PDT and PTT. The fluorescence of single QR is brighter and more stable than that of single QD. QRs may be more suitable for *in vivo* long-term fluorescent imaging.

Both semiconductor QDs and QRs are composed of heavy metal ions. Uncoated QDs or QRs such as CdTe exhibit highly toxicity to cell and animals, which have no prospect of clinical applications. For *in vivo* applications, QDs and QRs should be carefully coated with low or no toxic shells. Improving the qualities of QDs and QRs, such as improving the fluorescent quantum yield and photothermal conversion efficiency at NIR band, may be a good strategy for reducing the QD and QR toxicity to cells and animals since the toxicity of the QDs and QRs are dose dependent.

In this book, the QD and QR optical properties, SLN mapping, *in vivo* tumor target imaging, self-illuminating QDs for *in vivo* imaging, *in vivo* cancer PDT and PTT, as well as the QD-graphene nanosheet and QD-magnetic hybrid nanocomposites for bioimaging and cancer therapy were discussed. All contents besides the book cover were written and developed by Maoquan Chu, a Professor working at Tongji University in China. I hope this book will provide useful information on semiconductor QDs and QRs for *in vivo* fluorescent imaging and cancer phototherapy.

Prof. Maoquan Chu (储茂泉)
Research Center for Translational Medicine at Shanghai East Hospital, Tongji University, 150 Jimo Road, Shanghai 200120, P. R. China

and

School of Life Science and Technology, Tongji University Shanghai 200092, P. R. China
Email: mqchu98@tongji.edu.cn
May 3, 2015

About the Author

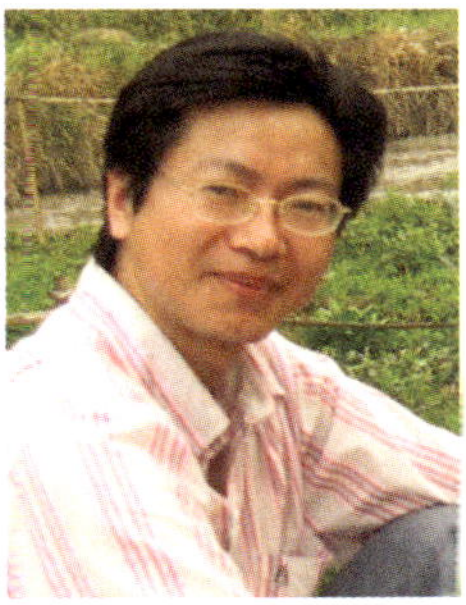

Professor Maoquan Chu was born in Anhui Province in China. He received his PhD in Chemical Engineering from East China University of Science and Technology in 2001. He then did his postdoctoral work in the School of Life Science and Technology in Shanghai Jiaotong University, where he delved into biomaterials and nanotechnology. In 2004, he attended the School of Life Science and Technology at Tongji University. In 2007, he won the China Education Ministry's "New Century Excellent Talents Supporting Plan". In 2008, he was hired as a Professor. He is now a principal investigator at the School of Life Science and Technology, Tongji University and also at the Research Center for Translational Medicine, Shanghai East Hospital in China. His main area of research is nanobiomedicine, with a current focus on cancer imaging and therapy using nanobiomaterials. His research work has been published in many important journals such as *Small*, *Biomaterials, Nanotoxicology*, *Theranostics*, *Nanoscale*, *Carbon*, etc.

Chapter 1

Semiconductor Quantum Dots for Sentinel Lymph Node Mapping through *In Vivo* Fluorescent Imaging

Semiconductor quantum dots (QDs) are nanocrystals that are just several nanometers in size, and therefore exhibit marked quantum size effects. Compared with organic dyes and fluorescent proteins, QDs possess interesting optical properties, including broad absorption, sharp size-tunable emission, high quantum yield and strong resistance to photobleaching. Since QDs were used as fluorescent nanoprobes for cell labeling and imaging in 1998, these fluorescent nanomaterials have been widely studied for *in vitro* and *in vivo* imaging applications. *In vivo* imaging using near-infrared (NIR) QDs shows potential for use in cancer diagnosis. Nanoparticles, including QDs, usually quickly accumulate in sentinel lymph nodes (SLNs) by passive targeting after being injected intramuscularly into a body. Therefore, using QD fluorescence for SLN mapping may be a convenient technique compared with other *in vivo* imaging applications such as tumor target imaging. Importantly, axillary SLNs containing NIR QDs can be imaged directly through deep tissue without surgical management, because the NIR fluorescence of such QDs can penetrate through tissue. In addition, the NIR fluorescence from the QDs in the SLNs can be observed for several hours or even longer. These advantages are benefit for SLN mapping. In this chapter, the optical properties of QDs and their use in animal SLN mapping are described. Future perspectives including the feasibility of clinical translation are also discussed.

1. Introduction

Semiconductor QDs, also called semiconductor metalloid-crystal nanostructures, are small nanoparticles that are usually spherical in shape, possess bulk-like crystalline structures and contain around 200–10,000 atoms. The size of QDs ranges from 1 to 10 nm, which is close to or smaller than the dimensions of the exciton Bohr radius. The most commonly used QDs in biomedical research are cadmium (Cd)-based, especially cadmium selenide (CdSe) and cadmium telluride (CdTe). The band gap, which is the energy difference between the top of the valence band and the bottom of the conduction band, of Cd-based QDs is located between 1.7 and 3.5 eV [1]. As a result, they emit bright visible (blue, green, yellow, or red) and near-infrared (NIR) fluorescence from a low energy band. For example, the fluorescent emission spectrum of CdSe QDs can extend to ~700 nm, and that of CdTe QDs can extend to ~800 nm [2, 3]. CdSe and CdTe QDs are easy to synthesize in aqueous solution, and the products obtained are water-soluble. They typically display fluorescence with a narrow full width at half-maximum (FWHM), short lifetime and high quantum yield. These features have facilitated the use of CdSe and CdTe QDs as well as those coated with an inorganic shell of zinc sulfide (ZnS) or silica in both *in vitro* and *in vivo* fluorescent imaging for biomedical detection.

However, Cd is a probable carcinogen, and has a long biological half-life in the body [4]. Therefore, Cd-free QDs have also attracted considerable worldwide attention recently. These Cd-free QDs include III(A)–V(A) semiconductors like indium arsenide and indium phosphide, IV(A)–VI(A) semiconductors such as lead selenide (PbSe) and lead sulfide, II(B)–VI(A) semiconductors including mercury telluride and zinc selenide, I(B)–VI(A) semiconductors such as silver sulfide and silver selenide, and I(B)–III(A)–VI(A) semiconductors including copper indium sulfide ($CuInS_2$) and copper indium selenide. The band gaps of most of these Cd-free QDs are narrower than those of the visible QDs mentioned above. For example, the band gaps of PbSe and lead telluride are less than 0.5 eV [5]. Therefore, such Cd-free QDs can be excited by visible and NIR photons and then emit NIR fluorescence from a low energy band [6]. However, these Cd-free QDs are usually synthesized in organic solution and their quantum yield obviously decreases when they are transferred into aqueous solution. In addition, most of these Cd-free QDs exhibit fluorescence with a broad FWHM, long lifetime and low quantum yield compared with that of Cd-based QDs [7].

The fluorescence of both Cd-containing and Cd-free QDs is superior to that of traditional organic dyes, which is the most attractive properties of QDs. Since QDs were first used for cell labeling and fluorescent imaging by Nie *et al.* [8] and Alivisatos *et al.* [9] in 1998, these novel fluorescent nanomaterials have attracted great attention in biomedical research for *in vivo* tissue-targeted imaging. SLN imaging using QDs may be the most easily achieved example of *in vivo* targeted imaging. This is because QDs passively migrate into lymph channels and then accumulate in SLNs after being injected subcutaneously into a body. In this chapter, the optical properties of QDs and their use in SLN mapping are described.

2. Optical Properties of QDs

Labeling and tracing of molecules or cells are very important techniques in biomedical research. Compared with radioactive tracers, fluorescent probes are less hazardous to animals and humans. Moreover, fluorescent imaging is simple and convenient. Semiconductor QDs can be used as ultra-sensitive fluorescent probes for *in vitro* and *in vivo* biomedical imaging because of their unique optical properties. Semiconductor QDs possess several advantages over traditional organic fluorescent dyes, fluorescent proteins, and lanthanide chelates as imaging probes, which are discussed as follows:

(1) QDs exhibit size-dependent fluorescence because of strong quantum confinement effects.

The optical properties of QDs can be tuned by changing their size because the band-gap energy of QDs is controlled by size. The larger the QDs, the lower their band-gap energy, which is termed the quantum confinement effect. As a result, large QDs can be excited by low-energy light, and then emit low-energy fluorescence; that is, at a long wavelength. Therefore, the color of fluorescent from QDs changes from blue

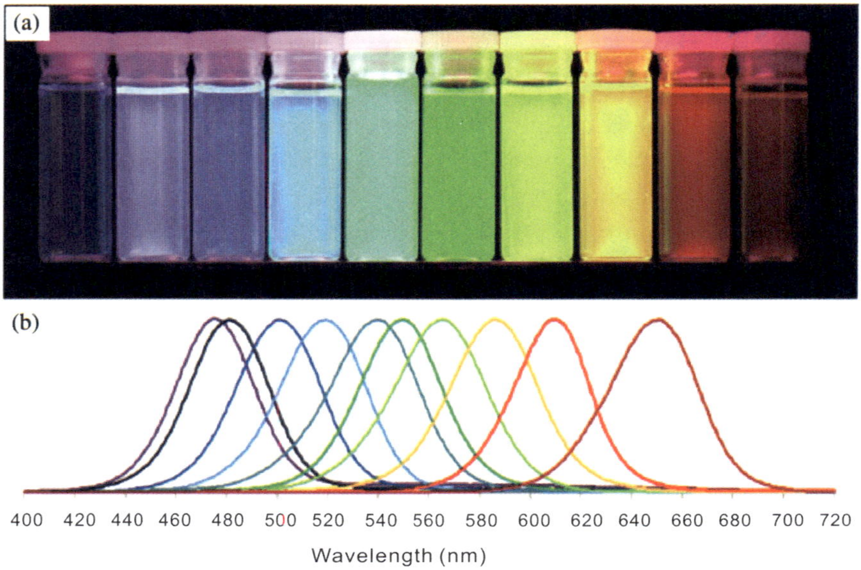

Fig. 1.1. Size-dependent optical properties of Cd-containing CdSe/ZnS QDs. (a) Fluorescent image of 10 vials of monodisperse QDs of different size. (b) Fluorescence spectra of the same 10 QD solutions. The fluorescent emission maxima are located at 443, 473, 481, 500, 518, 543, 565, 587, 610, and 655 nm (from left to right), respectively. Reprinted with permission from Ref. [10]. Copyright (2009) Elsevier.

to green, yellow, then red (including NIR) as their size increases. As shown in Fig. 1.1, as the diameter of CdSe/ZnS core–shell QDs increased slightly, their fluorescence obviously shifted to a longer wavelength. This was visibly observed as changes in the color of the QD solution [10]. QDs of the same materials that emit multiple colors are therefore easily obtained by tailoring their size, which is attractive for high-throughput biological detection. The color and intensity of QD fluorescence can also be varied by changing the composition or surface coating of the QDs. Figure 1.2 shows the distinct fluorescence of Cd-free $CuInS_2$/ZnS core–shell QDs with different diameters [11]. In addition, CdSe/ZnS QDs of the same diameter as $CuInS_2$/ZnS ones emit fluorescence of different colors.

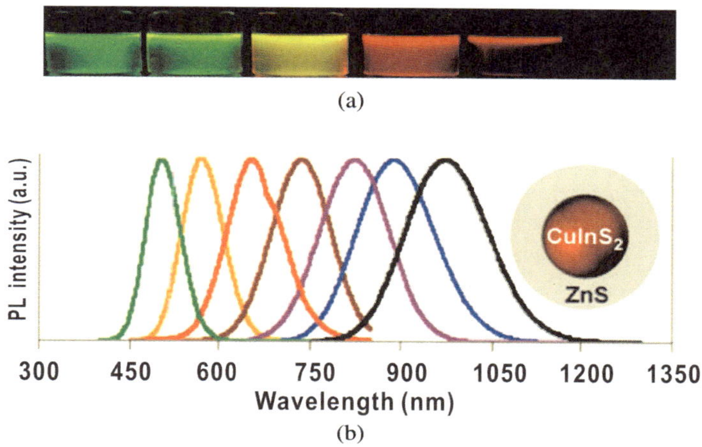

Fig. 1.2. Size-dependent optical properties of Cd-free $CuInS_2$/ZnS QDs. (a) Fluorescent images of monodisperse QDs of different size. (b) Fluorescence spectra of the same QD solutions. Reprinted with permission from Ref. [11]. Inset is a diagram of the structure of a single QD. Copyright (2009) American Chemical Society.

(2) QDs have broad continuous excitation spectra and narrow symmetric fluorescent emission spectra.

QDs exhibit broad continuous excitation spectra extending from ultraviolet to the NIR region (at shorter wavelength than that of emission). Therefore, QD fluorescence can be generated by a wide range of excitation wavelengths, and different-colored QDs can be excited simultaneously by a single light source. Figure 1.3a shows the broad absorption spectra of four sizes of CdSe QDs (2.2, 2.9, 4.1 and 7.3 nm) [12]. The absorption band edge of the largest QDs (7.3 nm) extends to longer than 650 nm. This is contrast to organic fluorescent materials, e.g., methylene blue (Fig. 1.3d) [13], which exhibit a sharp absorption spectrum. These four sizes of CdSe QDs display narrow symmetric fluorescence spectra, and their emission peaks are separated from each other (Fig. 1.3b) [12]. In addition, these QD solutions simultaneously emit bright blue, green, orange-red and deep red fluorescence when they are irradiated by a single ultraviolet source (Fig. 1.3c) [12].

In another example, the polymer coated CdSe/ZnS QD microbeads with a diameter of 0.5 μm that exhibited green, yellow and red

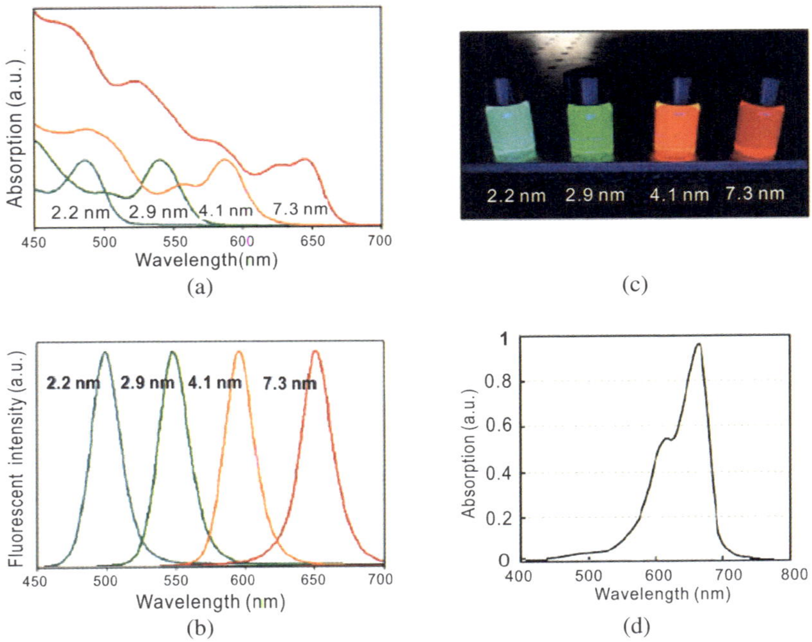

Fig. 1.3. Optical properties of different-sized CdSe QDs and methylene blue. (a) Absorption and (b) emission spectra of CdSe QDs. (c) True-color fluorescent images of CdSe QDs. (d) Absorption spectrum of methylene blue. The labels in (a)–(c) represent the respective diameters of the CdSe QDs. The images of (a), (b) and (c) were reprinted with permission from Ref. [12]. Copyright (2008) Elsevier. The image (d) was adapted with permission from Ref. [13], Copyright (2010) Elsevier.

fluorescence were injected subcutaneously at three adjacent locations in a host mouse. Wavelength-resolved spectral imaging was then carried out using a spectral imaging system (CRI, Inc., Woburn, MA, USA) composed of an optical head containing a liquid crystal tunable filter with a bandwidth of 20 nm and scanning wavelength range of 400–720 nm. Excitation of the QD microbeads caused them to simultaneously emit bright green, yellow, and red fluorescence (Fig. 1.4) [14]. These emission properties of QDs also can be seen in Figs. 1.1 and 1.2 above. Multiple-colored QD beads suitable for gene, protein and small-molecule library encoding [10, 15] have been developed because of the narrow emission and broad absorption spectra of QDs.

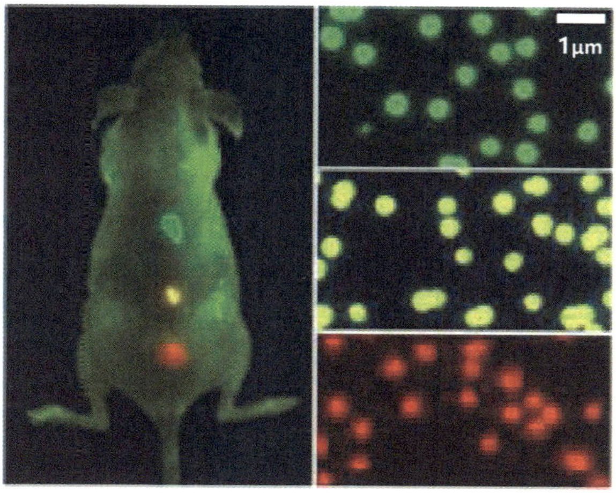

Fig. 1.4. Multicolor CdSe/ZnS-encoded fluorescent microbeads for simultaneous imaging. Left: a mouse was subcutaneously injected with CdSe/ZnS QD-encoded microbeads (0.5-μm diameter) emitting green, yellow or red light. Right: The true-color fluorescence of the three types of CdSe/ZnS QD-encoded microbeads. Reprinted with permission from Ref. [14]. Copyright (2004) Nature Publishing Group.

(3) High fluorescent quantum yield and photostability.

One of the main reasons why QDs have been widely used in biomedical research is that they exhibit both high fluorescent quantum yield and photostability. The very bright fluorescence of QDs helps to minimize the interference from background light during imaging. The quantum yield of high-quality QDs can reach up to 90%, which is much higher than that of traditional dyes. For example, the fluorescence of a single CdSe QD is 20 times brighter than that of a rhodamine 6G molecule [8]. High fluorescence stability helps researchers to study the dynamic process of a target objective over a long period, such as changes in the *in vivo* distribution of drugs over time, and the movement of proteins or drugs through cell membranes. The fluorescence of QDs can withstand extended irradiation. For example, the fluorescence bleaching rate of CdSe QDs is 100 times lower than that of rhodamine 6G [8]. Wu *et al.* [16] monitored the photostability of CdSe/ZnS QDs (emission peak: 630 nm) and organic fluorescent dye Alexa Fluor 488 in living cells (Fig. 1.5). Their results showed that the QDs in living 3T3 cells retained their strong fluorescence intensity.

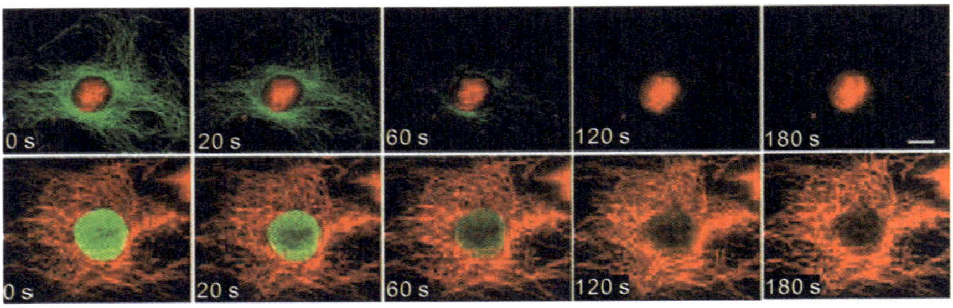

Fig. 1.5. Stability of red fluorescence from CdSe/ZnS QDs and green-organic fluorescence from Alexa 488, respectively, in living 3T3 cells. Reprinted with permission from Ref. [16]. Copyright (2003) Nature Publishing Group. (Note: top raw, QDs located in nucleus and Alexa 488 located in cytoplasm; bottom raw, QDs located in cytoplasm and Alexa 488 located in nucleus)

The fluorescent signal from QDs in the cells was stable against photobleaching, whereas Alexa 488 was bleached quickly. For the QD bioconjugates, the fluorescence intensity after 60 s of irradiation was 104% of the initial intensity for glycerol-mounted specimens. In contrast, the fluorescence intensity of Alexa 488 decreased to 50% of the initial intensity after 10 s, and 10% after 60 s.

Based on the unique optical properties described above, researchers have applied QDs in many fields of biology and medicine, especially in cell labeling, *in vivo* SLN mapping and tumor-targeted imaging.

3. QDs for SLN Mapping

3.1 SLNs and the importance of SLN detection

Lymph nodes (LNs) are small round organs that are dispersed throughout the body but primarily located in the neck, axilla, abdomen and groin. Many types of cancers spreading from the primary site to other organs usually flow through lymph vessels and LNs. The first node (or group of nodes) to receive lymphatic drainage from the primary tumor is the SLN. The relationship between the primary tumor and SLN(s) is illustrated in Fig. 1.6 [17]. If SLNs contain cancer cells, the cancer cells in the primary tumor may have migrated to other parts of the body (cancer metastases). Conversely, if SLNs are normal, the other LNs may be also normal, and the patient may be at an early stage of the disease. Therefore, SLN

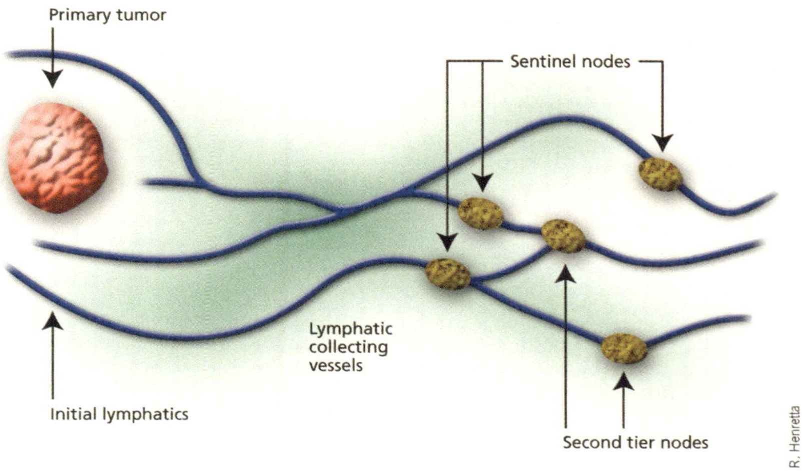

Fig. 1.6. Cancer spreading through the lymphatic system, and the positions of SLNs. Reprinted with permission from Ref. [17]. Copyright (2004) Nature Publishing Group.

mapping and biopsies are very important for determining the progress of cancer and the extent of surgical treatment.

3.2 NIR QDs for SLN mapping by *in vivo* fluorescent imaging

3.2.1 *The advantages of NIR QDs for SLN mapping over traditional techniques*

(1) Traditional techniques

In clinical practice, blue dye staining, radiocolloid tracer labeling, or a combination of both techniques are popular choices for patient SLN mapping. Blue staining is easily distinguished from the surrounding tissues, so blue-dyed SLNs are therefore convenient to observe and resect from the body. Methylene blue, isosulfan blue, Evans blue and patent blue are the most commonly used blue molecular dyes for SLN staining. However, LNs that have been dyed with these blue molecules cannot be directly observed except when the skin and muscle are incised, so a large wound is often unavoidable [18]. In addition, the blue dye molecules have a small hydrodynamic diameter; e.g., methylene blue has a diameter of only 0.7 nm and length of 1.6 nm [19]. As a result, dyes that have been trapped in the SLN usually flow to more distal nodes easily. Injection of a radiocolloid for SLN mapping is less invasive than staining with blue dye, but will expose the patient and surgeon to some radiation, which may be harmful [18]. Although blue staining and radiotracer imaging are often used synchronously to improve the level of SLN mapping, the limitations of these approaches are difficult to overcome.

(2) Advantages of NIR QDs for SLN mapping

Compared with the above traditional techniques, *in vivo* NIR fluorescent imaging using QDs has considerable advantages for SLN mapping.

First, NIR QDs have strong fluorescence intensity, so SLNs labeled with a low dosage of NIR QDs can be observed in real time without resecting skin and muscle to form a larger wound (Fig. 1.7). This is because NIR fluorescence strongly penetrates tissue, so it can be captured to allow highly sensitive *in vivo* imaging. For example, when a mouse was

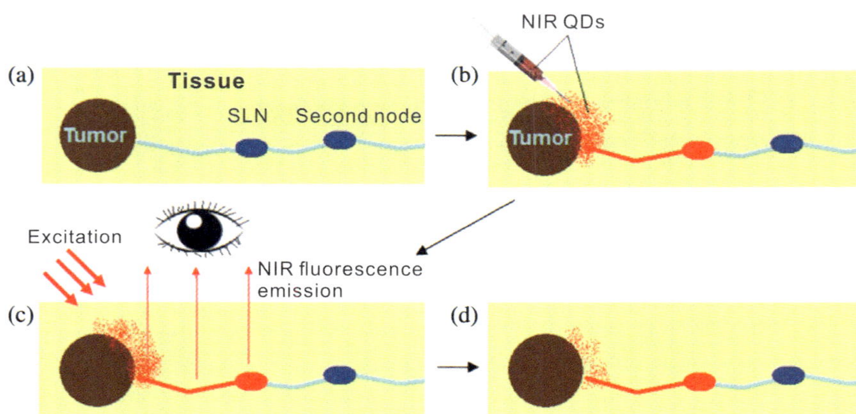

Fig. 1.7. Advantages of using NIR fluorescence of QDs for SLN mapping. (a) The tumor and nearby LNs. (b) NIR QDs migrate mainly into SLN after injection (c) Strong and relative stable NIR fluorescent signal generated by the QDs in deep tissue can be observed in real time without large surgical procedures. (d) NIR QDs locate in SLN for a long period due to the space resistance effect of the QDs. (The other two advantages described as following are not shown in this figure.)

injected intradermally with 10 pmol of NIR CdTe/CdSe core/shell QDs (hydrodynamic diameter: 15–20 nm; fluorescence emission: 840–860 nm) in a paw, and a pig (35 kg) was injected intradermally with 400 pmol of NIR QDs in a trotter, the SLNs in deep tissue (even 1 cm below the skin) could be imaged in real time through the tissue [20]. It should be noted that for a normal animal, SLN refers to the first LN or first group of LNs connecting the injection sites.

Second, NIR QDs have a larger hydrodynamic diameter and more stable fluorescence than most organic dyes, which allow operators to have enough time to accurately identify and resect SLNs because the QDs can be trapped by the SLNs and emit NIR fluorescence from the SLNs for a long period (Fig. 1.7). For example, when $CuInS_2$/ZnS QDs were subcutaneously injected into the right anterior paw of a mouse, the QDs rapidly migrated and accumulated in the corresponding SLN, and even at seven days post-injection the QDs in the SLN emitted bright fluorescence (Fig. 1.8) [21]. Interestingly, NIR QDs remained fluorescent even after 133 days in LNs [22], which originates from the suitable size and stable fluorescence of the QDs.

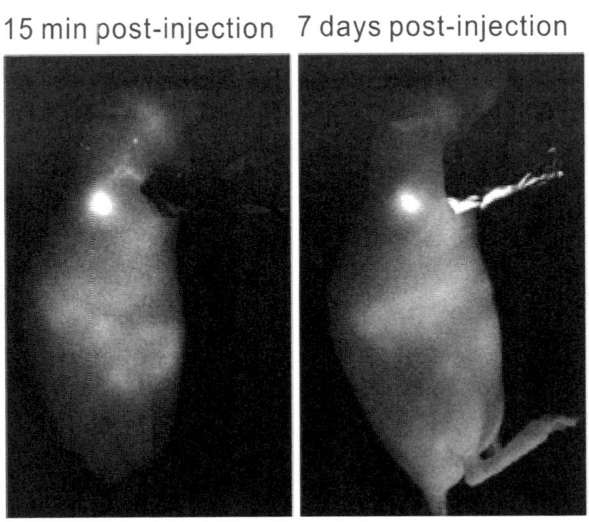

Fig. 1.8. Stability of NIR QDs in SLNs after subcutaneous injection. The mouse was injected with $CuInS_2$/ZnS QDs in the right anterior paw. Reprinted with permission from Ref. [21]. Copyright (2010) American Chemical Society.

It should be noted that QD hydrodynamic size plays an important role in their migration time through lymphatic vessels and LNs. A contrast agent with a size of 10–50 nm is ideal for SLN mapping [23, 24]. Larger particles usually remain at the injection site, while smaller particles (e.g., less than 5 nm) usually migrate into the blood stream after subcutaneous injection [25].

Third, different primary draining LNs in the body can be simultaneously imaged with QDs of different emission color. To assess lymphatic drainage from different separate drainage basins, traditional techniques such as X-ray lymphangiography and magnetic resonance (MR) lymphangiography require repeated separate study of each area [26]. This limitation of traditional techniques may be overcome by multicolor imaging using QDs. As mentioned above, fluorescence of different colors from QDs of different size can be simultaneously observed by excitation with a single light source. This optical property of QDs has great potential for independently identifying different tissues in a living body. In 2007, Kobayashi *et al.* [26] used three sizes of CdSe QDs with peak emission wavelengths of 565, 605 and 655 nm and two sizes of CdTe QDs with peak emission wavelengths of 705 and 800 nm for lymphatic multicolor imaging. They simultaneously injected one out of each of the five types of QDs intracutaneously into the middle phalanges, upper extremity, ears, and chin of a mouse (Fig. 1.9a). Wavelength-resolved spectral imaging was carried out using a spectral imaging system within 5 min of injection. Their results showed that all major drainage trunks (bilateral, superficial, deep cervical trunks, and trunks from bilateral upper extremities) of the lymphatics in the upper body of the mouse could be simultaneously visualized with different colors (Figs. 1.9b and 1.9c). This was the first demonstration of simultaneous imaging of five different lymphatic flows *in vivo* and their trafficking to distinct LNs.

Fourth, NIR fluorescence imaging does not require exposure to radiation, and has high resolution and sensitivity compared with those of radiotracers and dye absorption [27]. In addition, *in vivo* fluorescent imaging systems are cheaper than the instruments required by traditional techniques like computed tomography and MR imaging systems.

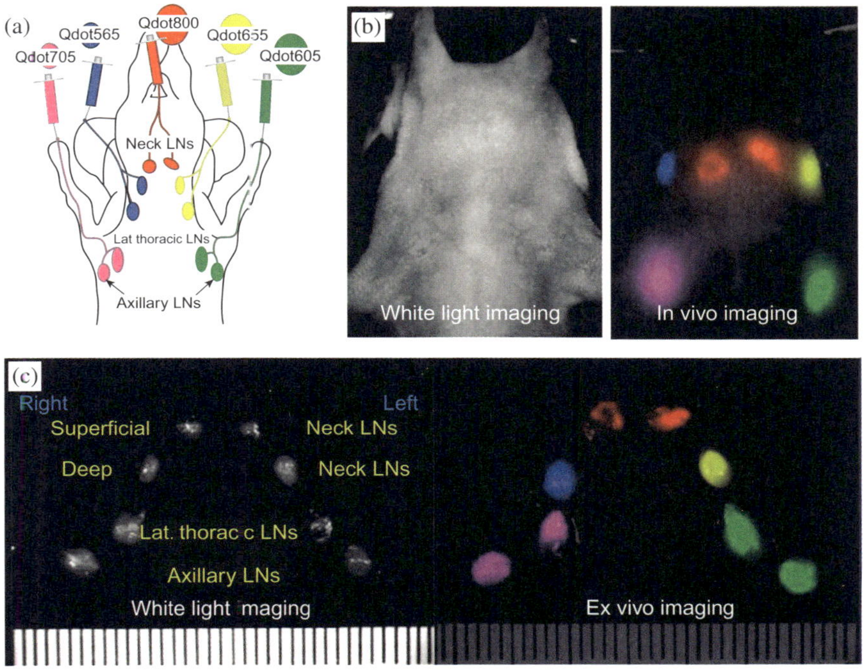

Fig. 1.9. Five distinct lymphatic drainage systems in the upper body of a mouse imaged using five types of QDs. (a) Schematic Illustration of QD injection sites and the corresponding primary draining LNs. (b) *In vivo* bright-field (left) and fluorescence (right) images of a mouse injected with QDs with different emission wavelengths. (c) Bright-field (left) and fluorescence (right) images of the eight draining LNs after surgical resection. Reprinted with permission from Ref. [26]. Copyright (2007) American Chemical Society.

3.2.2 *NIR QDs for mouse or rat SLN mapping*

In 2004, Kim *et al.* [20] first used oligomeric phosphine-coated CdTe/CdSe QDs (Fig. 1.10a) that emitted at 840–860 nm (called type-II QDs) with a quantum yield of ~13% for animal axillary SLN mapping. In type-II QDs, the electrons and holes are spatially separated between the core and shell to some extent, with the holes mostly confined to the core and the electrons having a preference for the shell (Fig. 1.10b), which causes type-II QDs to emit fluorescence of lower energy. When a mouse was

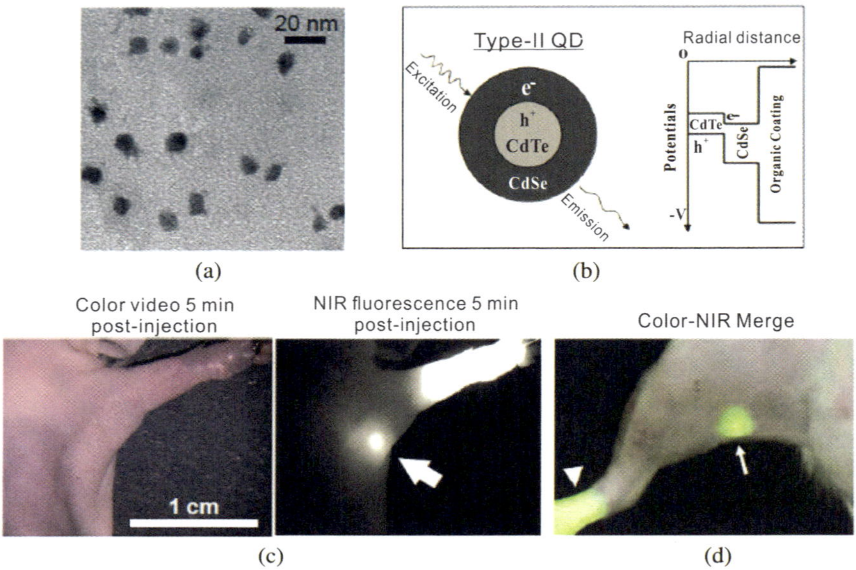

Fig. 1.10. (a) Transmission electron microscopy (TEM) image of oligomeric phosphine-coated CdTe/CdSe QDs dispersed in water. (b) Structure of type-II QDs (left) and potential diagram (right). (c) Images of a mouse after being intradermally injected with 10 pmol of the QDs in left front paw. (d) Image of a rat after being intradermally injected with 40 pmol of the QDs in a lower limb. Images of (a) and (c) were reprinted with permission from Ref. [20], Copyright (2003, 2007) Nature Publishing Group. Images of (b) and (d) were reprinted with permission from Ref. [28]. Copyright © 2007, Humana Press Inc., Totowa, NJ.

intradermally injected with such type-II NIR QDs in its left front paw, the NIR QDs entered the lymphatics and migrated rapidly to an axillary location. This process was clearly observed in real time through the fluorescence of the QDs using an *in vivo* imaging system (Fig. 1.10c). The axillary location was confirmed to be the SLN by a traditional method (mapping with isosulfan blue), because the blue dye also flowed to the same site.

Oligomeric phosphine-coated CdTe/CdSe core–shell QDs have also been used for SLN mapping of a lower limb of a rat. As shown in Fig. 1.10d, when a lower limb of a rat was injected with 40 pmol of these type-II QDs, NIR fluorescence imaging revealed fine details of the lymphatic flow from the injection site to the SLN of the limb [28].

The SLN containing NIR QDs in deep tissue can be accurately resected with the guidance of NIR fluorescence. In addition, surgeons would not require retraining to use this NIR QD mapping method because it is similar to the current intraoperative use of blue dye [17].

However, the potential toxicity of Cd in Cd-based QDs may prevent researchers from using such QDs in clinical SLN mapping. To lower the toxicity of QDs to animals during SLN mapping, Pons *et al.* [21] developed Cd-free $CuInS_2/ZnS$ QDs that emit NIR fluorescence for animal SLN imaging. To further lower the toxicity of the QDs and improve their water solubility, they encapsulated the $CuInS_2/ZnS$ QDs in phospholipid micelles, then used them for *in vivo* imaging and SLN mapping. After 20 pmol of the $CuInS_2/ZnS$ QDs was injected subcutaneously into the right anterior paw of a mouse, the right axillary LN could be easily visualized without surgery as early as a few minutes after injection (Fig. 1.11a), and the fluorescent signal detected in the LN increased with the injected dosage of QDs (Fig. 1.11b). To compare the toxicity of $CuInS_2/ZnS$ and CdTeSe/CdZnS QDs encapsulated in functionalized phospholipid micelles, Pons *et al.* subcutaneously injected 20 μL of each QD solution in the right anterior paws of different mice. They found that although the weight of the right axillary LNs increased with the injected dose of QDs because of the toxicity of the QDs, the same level of inflammation was caused by injection of 100 pmol of $CuInS_2/ZnS$ QDs or 10 pmol of CdTeSe/CdZnS QDs. Histological sections showed that the right axillary LN of mice injected with 20 pmol of $CuInS_2/ZnS$ had almost no obvious inflammation, whereas that of mice injected with the same dose of CdTeSe/CdZnS QDs were swollen and had inflammation sites (Fig. 1.11c).

3.2.3 *NIR QDs for SLN mapping in the groin, lung and esophagus of larger animals*

SLN mapping using QDs in large animal models may better resemble clinical practice than using rodents. In the past more than ten years, researchers have successfully introduced NIR QDs into pigs and dogs for SLN imaging. Kim *et al.* [20] found that when the thigh of a pig (35 kg)

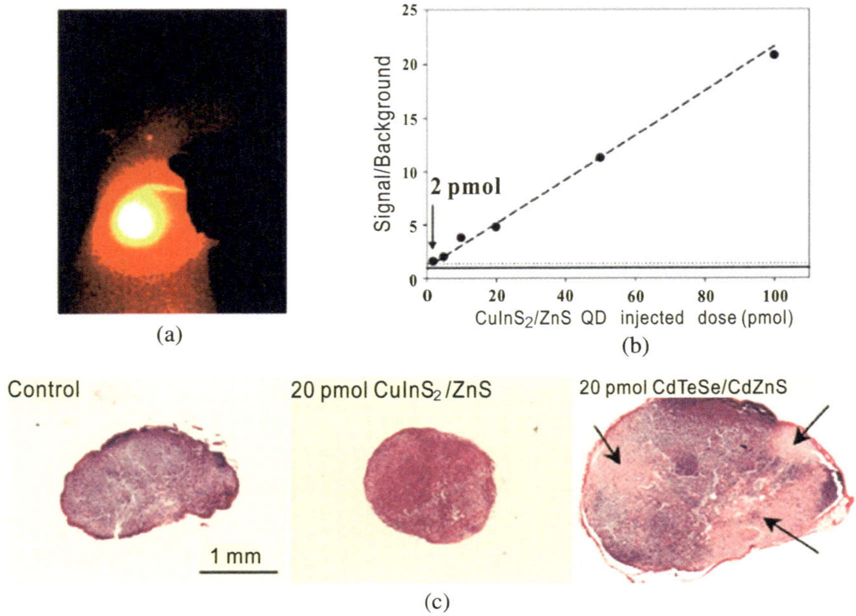

Fig. 1.11. (a) NIR fluorescence image of the right axillary LN of a mouse after subcutaneous injection of phospholipid micelle-encapsulated $CuInS_2$/ZnS core/shell QDs. (b) Ratio of the NIR fluorescence signal in the right axillary LN 24 h post-injection against autofluorescence background plotted as a function of the injected dose of $CuInS_2$/ZnS QDs. The solid line represents the autofluorescence background, and the dotted line represents the autofluorescence background plus three times the pixel-to-pixel standard deviation. (c) Histological sections of right axillary LNs resected seven days post-injection from mice injected with saline buffer solution (Control), 20 pmol of $CuInS_2$/ZnS QDs, and 20 pmol of CdTeSe/CdZnS QDs. The black arrows indicate inflammation sites. Reprinted with permission from Ref. [21]. Copyright (2010) American Chemical Society.

was injected intradermally with 400 pmol of oligomeric phosphine-coated CdTe/CdSe QDs, bright NIR fluorescence from the QDs migrated from the injection site to the SLN rapidly and a surgeon was able to follow lymphatic flow to quickly identify the position of the SLN (Fig. 1.12a). The SLN could be removed from the node field under the real-time visual guidance of the QDs (Figs. 1.12a and 1.12b). After the SLNs were resected from body, the SLN tissue and QD position were further confirmed by fluorescence imaging (Figs. 1.12c and 1.12d) [20].

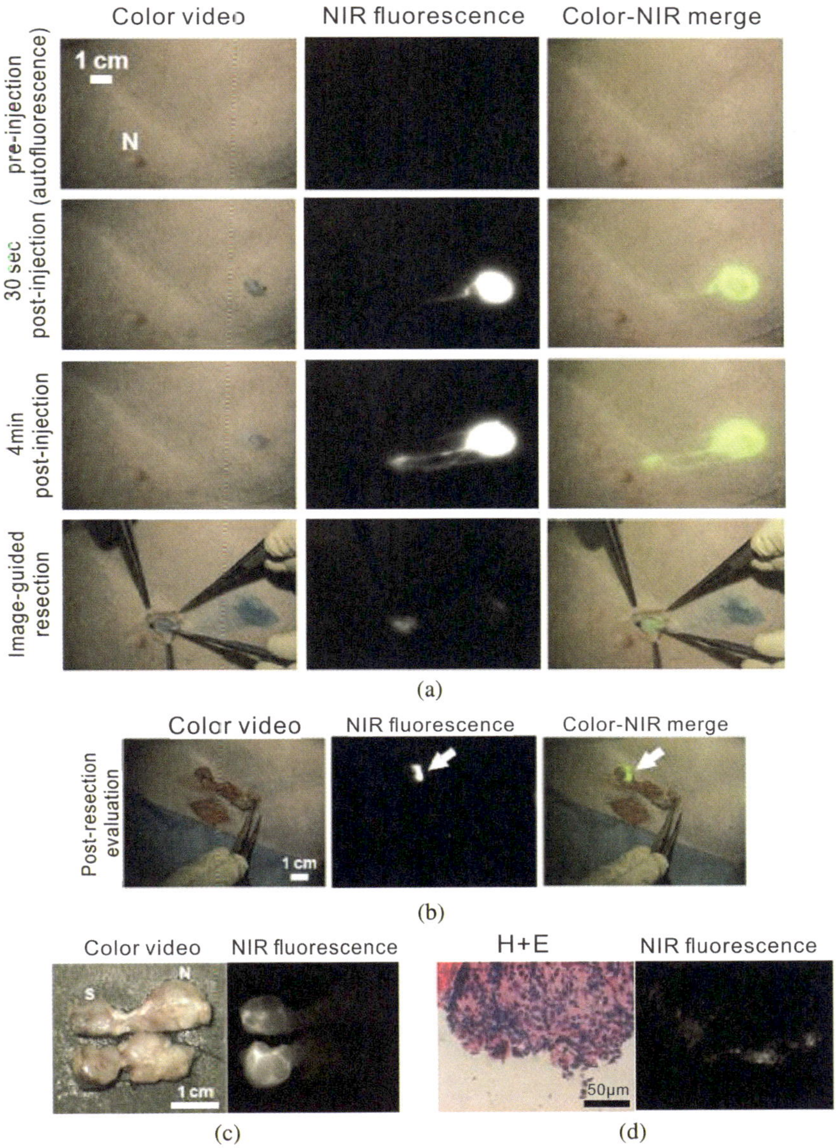

Fig. 1.12. Oligomeric phosphine-coated CdTe/CdSe type-II QDs used for SLN mapping in the groin of a pig. (a) Bright-field and corresponding NIR fluorescence images of the pig before and after injection of QDs. (b) Post-resection evaluation of the surgical field. (c) QD-labeled SLN (S) and the next LN (N) after resection. (d) Histologic analysis of hematoxylin and eosin (H&E)-stained sections of the QD-labeled SLN. Reprinted with permission from Ref. [20]. Copyright (2003) Nature Publishing Group.

In 2005, Soltesz *et al.* [29] used oligomeric phosphine-coated type-II CdTe/CdSe QDs with fluorescence emission at 840–860 nm to map pulmonary lymphatic drainage and guide excision of a SLN from a pig (mean weight 35 kg). They injected 200 pmol of NIR QDs ~1.5 cm deep into the medial surface of the right and left upper and lower lobes of the pig using a tuberculin syringe. Their results showed that the lymphatic pathway between the injection site and SLN could be observed. A LN emitted bright fluorescence just 45 s after injection, and no visible leakage of QDs from lymphatic vessels or nodal tissue was detected from the NIR fluorescent signal. After the QD-labeled SLN was resected and imaged, bright fluorescence could be clearly observed from this node compared with the adjacent nodal tissue. In addition, the NIR QDs were entrapped in the subcapsular and intermediate sinuses of the SLNs. This NIR QD mapping strategy could allow precise real-time imaging and overcome the limitations of traditional techniques. The results presented above indicate that NIR QDs could be used for SLN mapping of large animals with lung cancer.

NIR QDs can also be used for SLN mapping of the esophagus of large animals. For example, Parungo *et al.* [30] directly injected 200 pmol of oligomeric phosphine-coated CdTe/CdSe type-II QDs into the esophageal walls of pigs (mean weight 35 kg), then measured real-time fluorescence using an *in vivo* fluorescent imaging system. They found that a single SLN could be identified within 5 min in all of the injected pigs through the strong fluorescence signal from the QDs (Fig. 1.13a). In addition, *ex vivo* fluorescence and histologic photomicrographs further indicated that the SLN contained a large amount of NIR QDs compared with the control LN (Figs. 1.13b and 1.13c). Esophageal cancer is highly prevalent in China [31]. Surgical resection of early esophageal cancer is commonly used to prolong patient survival. SLN mapping using blue dye and/or radiocolloid tracer is typically used in esophageal cancer surgery. The level of esophageal cancer surgery may be improved in the future if NIR QDs with low toxicity are used for SLN mapping of human esophageal cancer.

3.2.4 *NIR QDs for tumor-bearing animal SLN mapping*

The SLN mapping using QD fluorescence described above was applied to healthy animals. In 2007, Ballou *et al.* [32] studied whether or not QDs

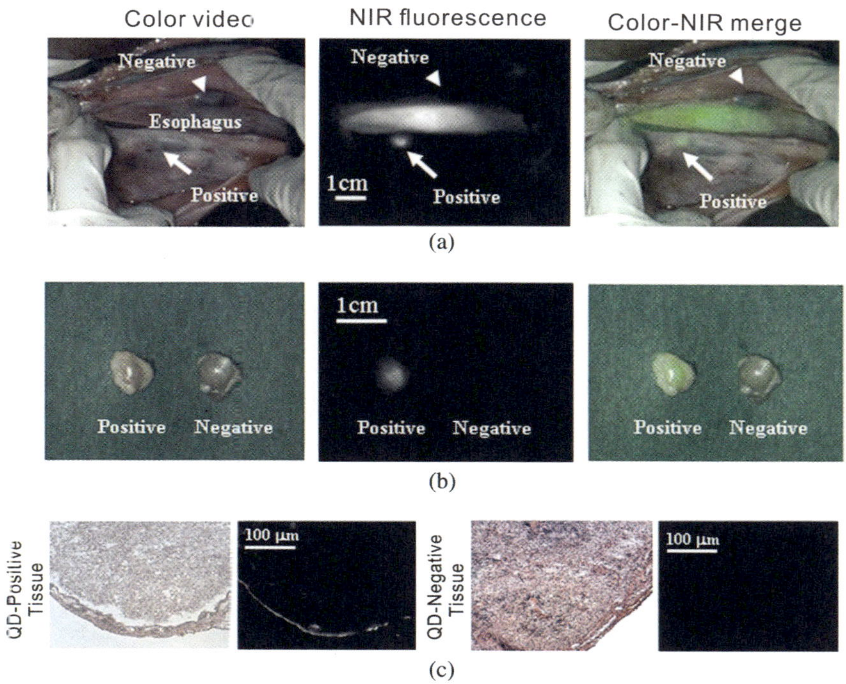

Fig. 1.13. Oligomeric phosphine-coated CdTe/CdSe type-II QDs used for SLN mapping of the esophagus of a pig. (a) Bright-field and corresponding NIR fluorescence images of the pig before and after injection of QDs. (b) QD-labeled SLN (left) and nearby negative nodes (right) after resection. (c) Histologic analysis of H&E-stained sections of the QD labeled SLN and control. Reprinted with permission from Ref. [30]. Copyright (2005) Elsevier.

could be injected into animal tumors to map tumor SLN. They used poly(ethylene glycol) (PEG)-coated CdSe/ZnS QDs with an emission wavelength of 655 nm and CdTe/CdSe/ZnS QDs with an emission wavelength of 800 nm for SLN mapping of mice with M21 melanoma and MH-15 teratocarcinoma, respectively. They found that QDs injected into the tumors rapidly migrated to SLNs, and there was no obvious difference in the QDs migrating from the tumor to surrounding LNs for PEG-coated QDs with terminal carboxyl, amino, and methoxyl groups, which was confirmed in real time through the fluorescence of the QDs. For example,

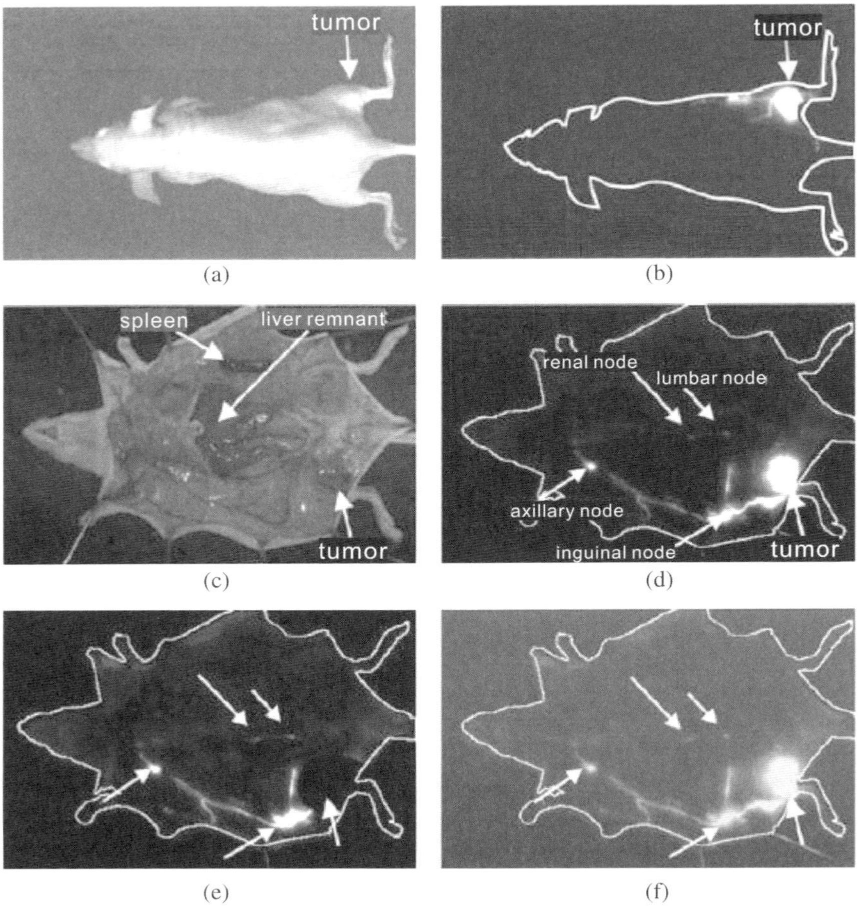

Fig. 1.14. PEG-COOH-coated CdSe/ZnS QDs for tumor SLN mapping of an M21 melanoma-bearing mouse. (a) Bright-field, and (b) *in vivo* fluorescent imaging at 655 nm. (c) Bright-field, and (d) *in vivo* fluorescent imaging at 655 nm of the mouse dissected 40 min post-injection. (e) Same as d, but with the tumor masked. (f) Same as d, but shown as a log-transformed image. Reprinted with permission from Ref. [32]. Copyright (2007) American Chemical Society.

after PEG-COOH-coated QDs (655-nm emission) were directly injected into a tumor (not into the surrounding tissue), fluorescence from the drainage system and SLN could be seen through the skin almost immediately after injection (Figs. 1.14a and 1.14b); drainage through the lymphatics to the right inguinal and axillary LNs, and migration of QDs to the right lumbar and renal nodes were also detected from the fluorescence of the QDs (Figs. 1.14c and 1.14f).

4. Discussion

Semiconductor QDs possess considerable advantages for *in vitro* and *in vivo* imaging such as tunable emission wavelength and high photostability, so many researchers have replaced organic fluorescent dyes with QDs for imaging studies. However, in practice, only high-quality QDs exhibit excellent optical properties compared with conventional fluorophores. Researchers need to have good knowledge of chemistry and materials science to synthesize high-quality QDs.

SLN biopsy can be used to quickly judge whether or not cancer cells have spread from the original tumor site. SLN mapping is an important part of SLN biopsy. Although the concept of SLN mapping is simple, it is usually difficult to perform accurately in a clinical setting [17]. Only the most experienced clinical doctors can rapidly identify the positions of SLN during surgery. Therefore, NIR QDs developed for SLN mapping using *in vivo* fluorescent imaging have attracted great attention from biomedical researchers. Following subcutaneous injection, NIR QDs can passively and quickly migrate to the SLN, allowing the SLN in deep tissue to be observed in real time through the NIR fluorescence of the QDs. These findings indicate that SLN mapping through *in vivo* fluorescence imaging using NIR QDs is a simple technique, and should not require surgeons with rich clinical experience. This is an advantage not only for doctors but also for patients, because less surgery is performed. The NIR QDs in SLNs emit bright, long-term fluorescence, so the surgeons can readily confirm that all the SLNs have been removed from the node field through real-time fluorescence guidance. In addition, NIR QDs are not radioactive and *in vivo* fluorescence imaging equipment is not expensive compared with other imaging equipment like that needed for X-ray imaging. It has been demonstrated that upon NIR laser irradiation, NIR QDs can convert laser light into heat energy [33–38]. Therefore, NIR QDs have potential for *in vivo* photothermal and photoacoustic imaging. If NIR fluorescence imaging is combined with photothermal or photoacoustic imaging, the accuracy of SLN mapping using NIR QDs may be improved compared with that of fluorescence imaging alone.

The route of administration for SLN mapping is local injection. After injection, some of the QDs remain at the injection site and in the SLN(s) for a long time. The toxicity of QDs administered through local injection may be obviously lower than that of QDs introduced though intravenous injection. However, the QDs are composed of heavy metals, and nanometer-sized QDs can penetrate through the intervals between cells. In early 2007, we found that when certain nanometer-sized CdTe QDs were coated on the hairless dorsal skin of mice, Cd atoms could be detected in the heart, liver, spleen, lung and kidney of the mouse [39]. Therefore, the toxicity and metabolism of QDs after local injection (e.g., subcutaneous injection) should be extensively studied before clinical translation. Use of NIR QDs for clinical SLN mapping will become possible only when low-toxicity QDs are developed.

References

[1] Murray CB, Sun SH, Gaschler W, Doyle H, Betley TA and Kagan CR. (2001). Colloidal synthesis of nanocrystals and nanocrystal superlattices. *Ibm. J. Res. Dev.*, **45**:47–56.

[2] Mahler B, Lequeux N and Dubertret B. (2010). Ligand-controlled polytypism of thick-shell CdSe/CdS nanocrystals. *J. Am. Chem. Soc.*, **132**:953–959.

[3] Rogach AL, Franzl T, Klar TA, Feldmann J, Gaponik N, Lesnyak V, Shavel A, Eychmculler A, Rakovich YP and Donegan JF. (2007). Aqueous synthesis of thiol-capped CdTe nanocrystals: State-of-the-art. *J. Phys. Chem. C.*, **111**:14628–14637.

[4] Henson MC and Anderson MB. (2000). The effects of cadmium on placental endocrine function. *Recent Res. Dev. Endocrinol.*, **1**:37–47.

[5] Wise FW. (2000). Lead salt quantum dots: the limit of strong quantum confinement. *Acc. Chem. Res.*, **33**:773–780.

[6] Pichaandi J and van Veggel FCJM. (2014). Near-infrared emitting quantum dots: Recent progress on their synthesis and characterization. *Coord. Chem. Rev.*, **263**:138–150.

[7] Cassette E, Helle M, Bezdetnaya L, Marchal F, Dubertret B and Pons T. (2013). Design of new quantum dot materials for deep tissue infrared imaging. *Adv. Drug Deliv. Rev.*, **65**:719–731.

[8] Chan WC and Nie S. (1998). Quantum dot bioconjugates for ultrasensitive nonisotopic detection. *Science*, **281**:2016–2018.

[9] Bruchez M, Moronne M, Gin P, Weiss S and Alivisatos AP. (1998). Semiconductor nanocrystals as fluorescent biological labels. *Science*, **281**:2013–2016.

[10] Zrazhevskiy P and Gao X. (2009). Multifunctional quantum dots for personalized medicine. *Nano Today*, **4**:414–428.

[11] Xie R, Rutherford M and Peng X. (2009). Formation of high-quality I-III-VI semiconductor nanocrystals by tuning relative reactivity of cationic precursors. *J. Am. Chem. Soc.*, **131**:5691–5697.

[12] Smith AM, Duan H, Mohs AM and Nie S. (2008). Bioconjugated quantum dots for *in vivo* molecular and cellular imaging. *Adv. Drug Deliv. Rev.*, **60**:1226–1240.

[13] Chu MQ and Wan YH. (2009). Sentinel lymph node mapping using near-infrared fluorescent methylene blue. *J. Biosci. Bioeng.*, **107**:455–459.

[14] Gao XH, Cui YY, Levenson RM, Chung LWK and Nie SM. (2004). *In vivo* cancer targeting and imaging with semiconductor quantum dots. *Nat. Biotechnol.*, **22**:969–976.

[15] Gao XH and Nie SM. (2004). Quantum dot-encoded mesoporous beads with high brightness and uniformity: Rapid readout using flow cytometry. *Anal. Chem.*, **76**:2406–2410.

[16] Wu XY, Liu HJ, Liu JQ, Haley KN, Treadway JA, Larson JP, Ge N, Pcale F and Bruchex MP. (2003). Immunofluorescent labeling of cancer marker Her2 and other cellular targets with semiconductor quantum dots. *Nat. Biotechnol.*, **21**:41–46.

[17] Uren RF. (2004). Cancer surgery joins the dots. *Nat. Biotechnol.*, **22**:38–39.

[18] Chu MQ, Xiao XA, Ma JY, Ji AL, Yuan RQ, Yang H, *et al.* (2010). *In vivo* real-time near-infrared fluorescent mapping of sentinel lymph nodes using methylene blue encapsulated in a microemulsion nanosystem. *Curr. Nanosci.*, **6**:388–396.

[19] Song KH, Kim CH, Cobley CM, Xia YN and Wang LV. (2009). Near-infrared gold nanocages as a new class of tracers for photoacoustic sentinel lymph node mapping on a rat model. *Nano Lett.*, **9**:183–188.

[20] Kim S, Lim YT, Soltesz EG, De Grand AM, Lee J, Nakayama A, Parker JA, Mihaljevic T, Laurence RG, Dor DM, Cohn LH, Bawendi MG and Frangioni JV. (2004). Near-infrared fluorescent type II quantum dots for sentinel lymph node mapping. *Nat. Biotechnol.*, **22**:93–97.

[21] Pons T, Pic E, Lequeux N, Cassette E, Bezdetnaya L, Guillemin F, Marchal F and Dubertret B. (2010). Cadmium-free CuInS2/ZnS quantum

dots for sentinel lymph node imaging with reduced toxicity. *Acs. Nano.*, **4**:2531–2538.

[22] Ballou B, Lagerholm BC, Ernst LA, Bruchez MP and Waggoner AS. (2004). Noninvasive imaging of quantum dots in mice. *Bioconjugate Chem.*, **15**:79–86.

[23] Josephon L, Mahmood U, Wunderbaldinger P, Tang Y and Weissleder Y. (2003). Pan and sentinel lymph node visualization using a near-infrared fluorescent probe. *Mol. Imaging*, **2**:18–23.

[24] Ohnishi S, Lomnes SJ, Laurence RG, Gogbashian A, Mariani G and Frangioni JV. (2005). Organic alternatives to quantum dots for intraoperative near-infrared fluorescent sentinel lymph node mapping. *Mol. Imaging*, **4**:172–181.

[25] Alazraki NP, Eshima D, Eshima LA, Herda SC, Murray DR, Vansant JP and Taylor AT. (1997). Lymphoscintigraphy, the sentinel node concept, and the intraoperative gamma probe in melanoma, breast cancer, and other potential cancers. *Semin. Nucl. Med.*, **27**:55–67.

[26] Kobayashi H, Hama Y, Koyama Y, Barrett T, Regino CAS, Urano Y and Choyke PL. (2007). Simultaneous multicolor imaging of five different lymphatic basins using quantum dots. *Nano Lett.*, **7**:1711–1716.

[27] Nune SK, Gunda P, Majeti BK, Thallapally PK and Forrest ML. (2011). Advances in lymphatic imaging and drug delivery. *Adv. Drug Deliv. Rev.*, **63**:876–885.

[28] Frangioni JV, Kim SW, Ohnishi S, Kim S and Bawendi MG. (2007). Sentinel lymph node mapping with type-II quantum dots. *Methods Mol. Biol.*, **374**:147–159.

[29] Soltesz EG, Kim S, Laurence RG, DeGrand AM, Parungo CP, Dor DM Cohn LH, Bawendi MG, Frangioni JV and Mihaljevic T. (2005). Intraoperative sentinel lymph node mapping of the lung using near-infrared fluorescent quantum dots. *Ann. Thorac Surg.*, **79**:269–277.

[30] Parungo CP, Ohnishi S, Kim SW, Kim S, Laurence RG, Soltesz EG, Chen FY, Colson YL, Cohn LH, Bawendi MG and Frangioni JV. (2005). Intraoperative identification of esophageal sentinel lymph nodes with near-infrared fluorescence imaging. *J. Thorac Cardiovasc Surg.*, **129**:844–850.

[31] Li LB, Xie JM, Zhang XN, Chen JZ, Luo YL, Zhang LY and Luo RC. (2010). Retrospective study of photodynamic therapy vs photodynamic therapy combined with chemotherapy and chemotherapy alone on advanced esophageal cancer. *Photodiagn. Photodyn Ther.*, **7**:139–143.

[32] Ballou B, Ernst LA, Andreko S, Harper T, Fitzpatrick JAJ, Waggoner AS and Bruchez MP. (2007). Sentinel lymph node imaging using quantum dots in mouse tumor models. *Bioconjug. Chem.*, **18**:389–396.

[33] Liu XJ, Li B, Fu F, Xu KB, Zou RJ, Wang Q, Zhang B, Chen Z and Hu J. (2014). Facile synthesis of biocompatible cysteine-coated CuS nanoparticles with high photothermal conversion efficiency for cancer therapy. *Dalton Trans.*, **43**:11709–11715.

[34] Li WH, Zamani R, Gil PR, Pelaz B, Ibanez M, Cadavid D, Shavel A, Alvarzy-Puebla RA, Parak WJ, Aribol J and Cabot A. (2013). CuTe nanocrystals: shape and size control, plasmonic properties, and use as SERS probes and photothermal agents. *J. Am. Chem. Soc.,* **135**:7098–7101.

[35] Chu MQ, Pan XJ, Zhang D, Wu Q, Peng JL and Hai WX. (2012). The therapeutic efficacy of CdTe and CdSe quantum dots for photothermal cancer therapy. *Biomaterials*, **33**:7071–7083.

[36] Hessel CM, Pattani VP, Rasch M, Panthani MG, Koo B, Tunnell JW and Korgel BA. (2011). Copper selenide nanocrystals for photothermal therapy. *Nano Lett.*, **11**:2560–2566.

[37] Tian QW, Tang MH, Sun YG, Zou RJ, Chen ZG, Zhu M, Yang S, Wang J and Hu J. (2011). Hydrophilic flower-like CuS superstructures as an efficient 980 nm laser-driven photothermal agent for ablation of cancer cells. *Adv. Mater.*, **23**:3542–3547.

[38] Li YB, Lu W, Huang QA, Huang MA, Li C and Chen W. (2010). Copper sulfide nanoparticles for photothermal ablation of tumor cells. *Nanomedicine (UK)*, **5**:1161–1171.

[39] Chu MQ, Wu Q, Wang JX, Hou SK, Miao Y, Peng JL, *et al.* (2007). *In vitro* and *in vivo* transdermal delivery capacity of quantum dots through mouse skin. *Nanotechnology*, **18**(45):5103 1–5106.

Chapter 2

Semiconductor Quantum Dots for *In Vivo* Tumor-targeted Imaging

In vivo tumor-targeted fluorescent imaging is a particularly promising method for real-time detection of solid tumors located in a body. This is a convenient and inexpensive technique compared with traditional imaging methods such as magnetic resonance and computed tomography imaging. *In vivo* tumor-targeted fluorescent imaging requires fluorescent agents that exhibit bright stable near-infrared (NIR) fluorescence and high tumor-targeting efficiency. High-quality NIR semiconductor quantum dots (QDs) covalently conjugated with biorecognition molecules like antibodies are excellent candidates as fluorescent agents because of their small size and high fluorescent quantum yield and photostability. In this chapter, *in vivo* passive and active tumor targeting of QDs, as well as the trajectory of tumor-targeted delivery of a single QD bioconjugate in live mice, are described.

1. Introduction

In Chapter 1, we described the optical properties of semiconductor QDs. QDs are inorganic fluorescent nanocrystals range in size from 1 to ~10 nm. The fluorescence of QDs is brighter and more stable than that of common organic dyes, fluorescent proteins and lanthanide chelates. An interesting optical property of QDs is their relationship between fluorescent color and size. The emission color of QDs can be fine-tuned from blue through green, yellow and red to NIR by increasing their size [1] and controlling their composition.

NIR emission is ideal for *in vivo* biomedical fluorescent imaging because NIR light can penetrate deep tissue and NIR imaging has a lower ratio of florescence signal to background (or noise) than other wavelengths. Therefore, QDs that emit NIR fluorescence are usually used for *in vivo* tumor-targeted imaging. Red QDs with emission ranging from 600 to 700 nm have also been used for *in vivo* detection in small animal models. Current NIR and red QDs reported for *in vivo* cancer targeting include cadmium selenide (CdSe)/zinc sulfide (ZnS) QDs that emit at 625 nm [2] and around 630–640 nm [3], CdSe/cadmium sulfide (CdS)/ZnS QDs rods with an emission maximum at 658 nm [4], cadmium telluride (CdTe)/CdS QDs with an emission maximum at 628 nm [5], CdTe/zinc selenide (ZnSe) QDs with an emission maximum at 730 nm [6], copper indium sulfide ($CuInS_2$)/ZnS QDs that emit in the range of 550–800 nm [7], lead selenide (PbSe) QDs with an emission maximum at 860 nm [8], and silver sulfide QDs with an emission maximum at ~1200 nm [9], etc. These QDs are often modified with polyethylene glycol (PEG) or other polymers, or coated with liposomes. To improve the efficiency of tumor targeting, the modified QDs are further conjugated with an antibody, ligand or peptide, or coated with bacteria and then conjugated with antibody. Schematic diagrams of the structures of commonly used PEG-coated QDs and functionalized QDs for *in vivo* targeted imaging are shown in Fig. 2.1 [10]. The *in vivo* targeting efficiency of these QD-based materials mainly depends on the ability of biorecognition molecules (e.g., antibody) to bind specifically to cancer cells, QD size, QD surface charge and the dispersion of QDs in animal blood. However, the fluorescent intensity of NIR QDs may decrease obviously when the QDs circulate in blood. Therefore, only NIR QDs with high fluorescent quantum yield and high tumor-targeting efficiency can efficiently light up an animal tumor with their NIR fluorescence after intravenous injection. *In vivo* tumor-targeted fluorescent imaging is a simple and

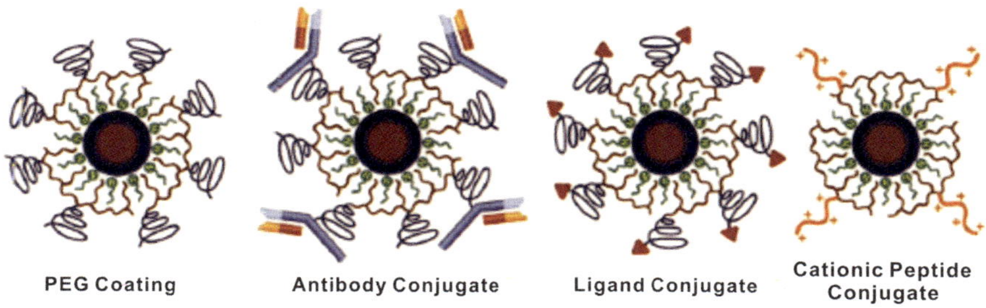

Fig. 2.1. Schematic diagrams of PEG-coated and bioconjugated QD fluorescent probes. Reprinted with permission from Ref. [10]. Copyright (2008) Elsevier.

convenient technique to identify where a tumor is located in an animal body in real time.

2. Tumor-targeted Imaging using QDs based on the Enhanced Permeability and Retention Effect

2.1 Enhanced permeability and retention effect in solid tumors

The organization of the microvasculature within tumor tissue is different from that of the microvasculature within normal tissue. In 1986, Maeda *et al.* [11] first presented the concept of an enhanced permeability and retention (EPR) effect in tumors. They found that many macromolecules (proteins) progressively accumulated in the tumor tissues of the mice after intravenous injection, and they speculated that this phenomenon may be related to the hypervasculature and enhanced permeability to macromolecules of the tumors, as well as little recovery through either blood vessels or lymphatic vessels. The EPR effect is the phenomenon that macromolecules or nanoparticles of certain sizes can readily penetrate into tumor tissue and accumulate more in tumors than in normal tissues, and also that the macromolecules or nanoparticles stay in the tumor for a longer time than small molecules. Since its proposal in 1986, the EPR effect has been widely confirmed by many researchers. For example, Skinner *et al.* [12]

found that in normal tissue, venules pass to submucosal veins without receiving further branches through the mucosa, and the capillaries within the mucosa are arranged in a regular honeycomb-like pattern around the mucosal glands. Conversely, tumor tissue contains many vessels that are irregular in shape and of greater density than normal. The disordered vasculature structure in tumors is characterized principally by variations in the size and direction of vessels, and increased numbers of interconnections without a perceptible pathway of flow. Tumor blood vessels can also be leaky or defective, and large fenestrations can be found between the endothelial cells [13]. This specific structure of tumor blood vessels can allow macromolecules or nanoparticles to migrate into tumor tissue through the vessel walls. Furthermore, after the macromolecules or nanoparticles are entrapped in the tumor tissue, they are retained in the tumor for a long period because of the slow venous return and poor lymphatic clearance in tumor tissue.

The EPR effect is an important mechanism for passive targeting of *in vivo* solid tumors with drugs or nanoparticles. Figure 2.2 shows the difference between small-molecule and macromolecular drugs passing through tumor blood vessels [13]. Small molecules can penetrate through the

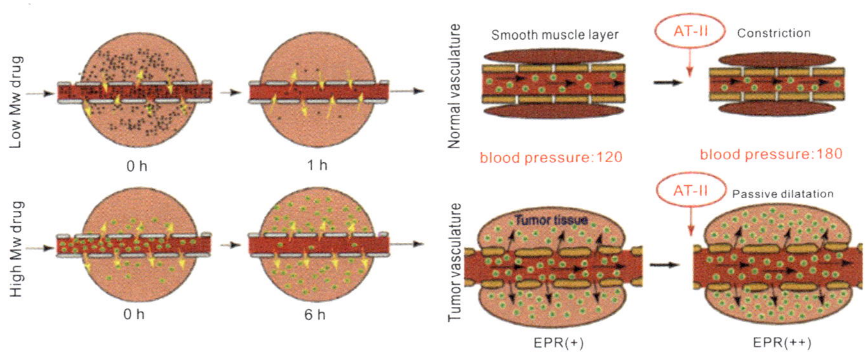

Fig. 2.2. Diagrammatic representation of the EPR effect. (a) Diffusion of drugs with low molecular weight (Mw) (black spots) and high Mw (green spots with yellow circles) from the blood vessels into the interstitium of tumor tissue (large pink circles). (b) Illustration of vascular leakage in response to angiotensin-II (AT-II)-induced hypertension and the subsequent contraction of the smooth muscle layer. The absence of a smooth muscle layer in tumor blood vessels leads to enhanced extravasation of macromolecular drugs and thus augments the EPR effect. Reprinted with permission from Ref. [13]. Copyright (2006) Elsevier.

normal blood vessel. Small molecules can also penetrate through (pass in and out) tumor blood vessel walls more easily than the larger ones, so the effective concentration of smaller molecules in the tumor is obviously lower than that of larger ones after one or several hours of blood circulation (Fig. 2.2a). Angiotensin-II can cause a selective increase in tumor blood flow volume, and the hypertensive state induced by this exogenous agent can augment the EPR effect. This allows more macromolecular drugs to diffuse into the tumor tissue through abnormal blood vessels (Fig. 2.2b). The information presented in Fig. 2.2 demonstrates the importance of the EPR effect in *in vivo* tumor-targeted drug delivery.

2.2 Passive targeting of tumor tissue by QDs

QDs exhibit excellent optical properties, so these nanomaterials have great potential for *in vivo* solid tumor diagnosis or confirming that drugs have been delivered to tumor sites by *in vivo* fluorescent imaging. To achieve this, the QDs need to successfully penetrate through many barriers (e.g., the reticuloendothelial system) *in vivo* and finally migrate to the tumor tissue. However, after intravenous injection or oral administration, nanoparticles usually tend to be nonspecifically captured by the liver, spleen, lung, and other organs, so only a small amount of nanoparticles arrives at the tumor site. To reduce this, the QD surface will be coated with a polymer, typically PEG. PEG modification can markedly reduce the uptake of QDs by the reticuloendothelial system and avoid rapid renal filtration.

To further improve the tumor-targeting efficiency of PEG-coated QDs, Al-Jamal *et al.* [14] encapsulated cadmium-containing NIR QDs into micelles composed of functionalized PEG (Lipid-PEG-COOH). These PEGylated lipid-coated QDs (functionalized QDs, abbreviated as *f*-QDs) were then embedded in cationic liposome vesicles formed from dioleoylphosphatidylcholine, cholesterol (Chol) and 1,2-dioleoyl-3-trimethylammoniumpropane (DOTAP) or embedded in PEGylated liposome vesicles (PEGylated lipid layer-coated f-QDs, abbreviated as *f*-QDs-L). They then injected the *f*-QD or *f*-QD-L hybrids (200 μL, 33 pmol of *f*-QD) into B16F10 melanoma tumor-bearing C57BL6 mice via tail veins. The cationic liposome-coated *f*-QDs exhibited faster blood clearance and higher liver uptake than PEGylated *f*-QD-L hybrid vesicles. In addition,

PEGylated *f*-QD-L hybrid vesicles accumulated in the tumor lesions much more rapidly than *f*-QD, and were retained in the tumor for at least 24 h. It should be noted that these modified NIR QDs were not conjugated with any antibodies, peptides or other ligands. The rapid accumulation of the *f*-QD-L hybrids in the tumor after intravenous injection is mainly related to the EPR effect.

Shuhendler *et al.* [8] encapsulated NIR PbSe QDs into fatty ester nanoparticles (FEN) and then the QD-FEN were coated with PEG chains (Fig. 2.3). They injected 200 μL of a saline suspension of PEG-QD-FENs (64 μg of PbSe QDs in total) into the tail veins of mice bearing breast tumors grown from the MDA-435 cell line to perform tumor-targeted imaging using the QDs. They observed tumor fluorescence above tissue background 30 min after intravenous administration (Fig. 2.4a). The fluorescent intensity of the tumor 60 or 120 min post-injection was brighter than that at 30 min post-injection. The tumor still emitted fluorescence 3 h after PEG-QD-FEN injection, which could be observed in real time by

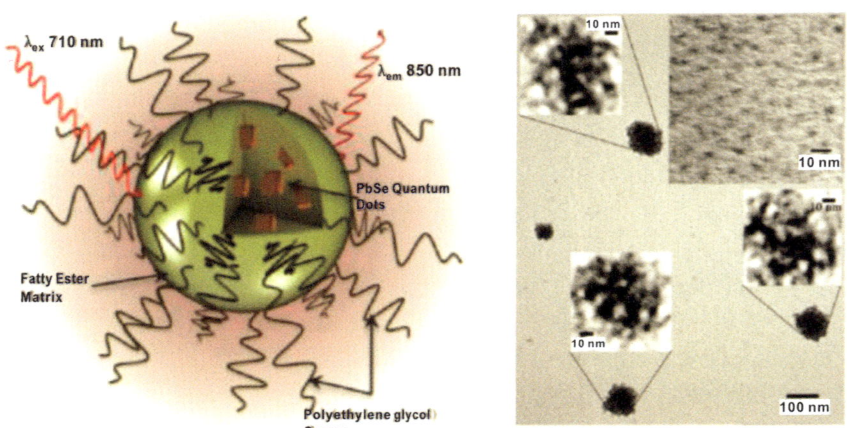

(a) (b)

Fig. 2.3. (a) Schematic diagram of PbSe QDs being dispersed throughout the FEN matrix and modified with PEG. (b) Transmission electron microscopy (TEM) images of PEG-QD-FENs (top right inset: PbSe QDs). Reprinted with permission from Ref. [8]. Copyright (2011) American Chemical Society.

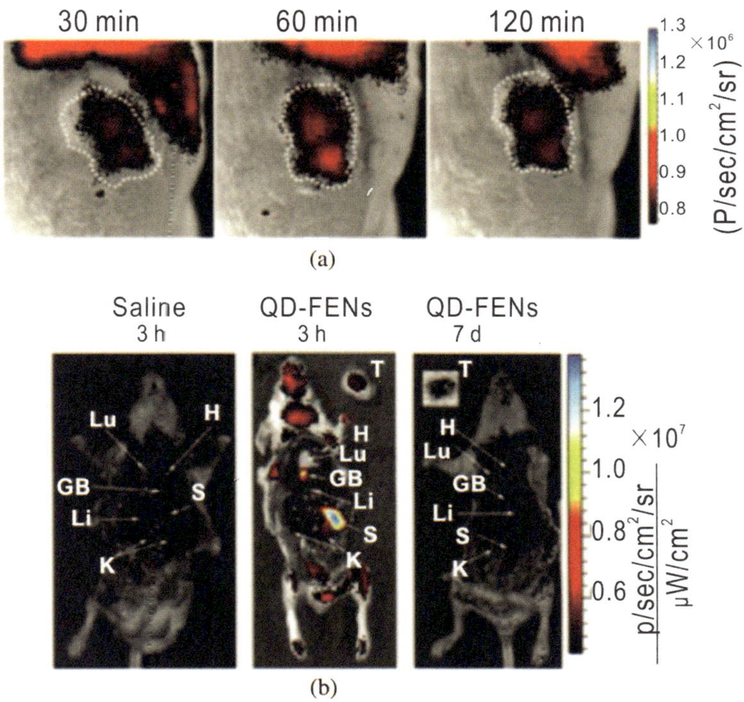

Fig. 2.4. *In vivo* fluorescent images of mice bearing breast tumors after intravenous injection with PEG-QD-FENs and control. (a) Tumor accumulation of the PEG-QD-FENs was noted 30, 60 and 120 min after intravenous administration. (b) Necropsy analysis of the tissue distribution showed considerable accumulation of PEG-QD-FENs in the spleen and gall bladder, without accumulation in the liver, after 3 h. Near complete elimination of the PEG-QD-FENs was observed seven days after administration. GB, gall bladder; H, heart, K, kidney; Li, liver; Lu, lung; S, spleen; T, tumor. Reprinted with permission from Ref. [8]. Copyright (2011) American Chemical Society.

in vivo fluorescent imaging (Fig. 2.4b). In addition, the PEG-QD-FENs may be cleared from the mouse body, which was also confirmed by *in vivo* imaging (Fig. 2.4b). This hybrid nanoparticulate fluorophore system also has no conjugated antibody, peptide or ligand. Instead, the passive delivery of the PEG-QD-FEN fluorescent probes to tumor tissue may be also mainly caused by the EPR effect.

3. Antibody-conjugated QDs for *In Vivo* Tumor-targeted Imaging

Although it has been demonstrated that QDs can passively accumulate in tumor tissue, in some cases the NIR fluorescence in tumor tissue was difficult to detect because of low targeting efficiency of the QDs. Therefore, QDs are often conjugated with tumor-targeting ligands such

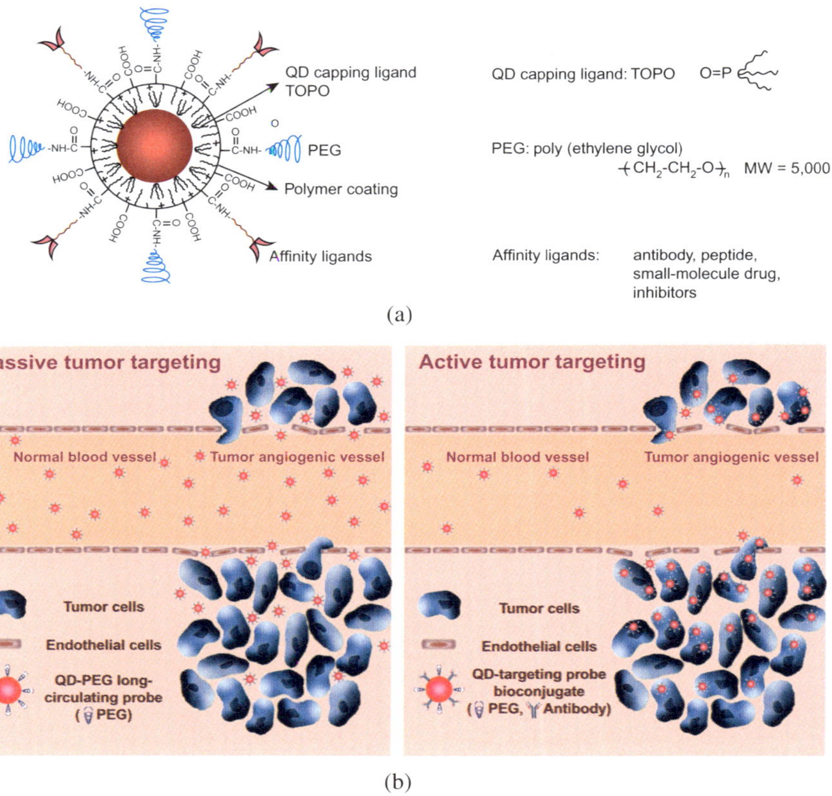

Fig. 2.5. (a) Structure of a multifunctional QD probe, showing the capping ligand tri-*n*-octylphosphine oxide (TOPO), an encapsulating copolymer layer, tumor-targeting ligands (such as peptides, antibodies or small molecule inhibitors) and PEG. (b) Permeation and retention of QD probes via passive targeting (left) and active targeting (right). Reprinted with permission from Ref. [3]. Copyright (2004) Nature Publishing Group.

as antibodies and peptides to improve their tumor-targeting efficiency (Fig. 2.5a) [3]. These bioconjugated QDs migrate to tumor sites through both leaky tumor vasculature (passive targeting) and the strong affinity binding of QD conjugates to tumor antigens (active targeting) (Fig. 2.5b). After the QD bioconjugates recognize the tumor cell surfaces, QDs strongly adhere to the cancer cells. In addition, QD bioconjugates may further migrate into cancer cells via endocytosis. These may be the main reasons that active targeting is much more efficient than passive targeting.

In 2004, Gao *et al.* [3] conjugated amphiphilic triblock polymer and a tumor-targeting ligand, prostate-specific membrane antigen (PSMA)

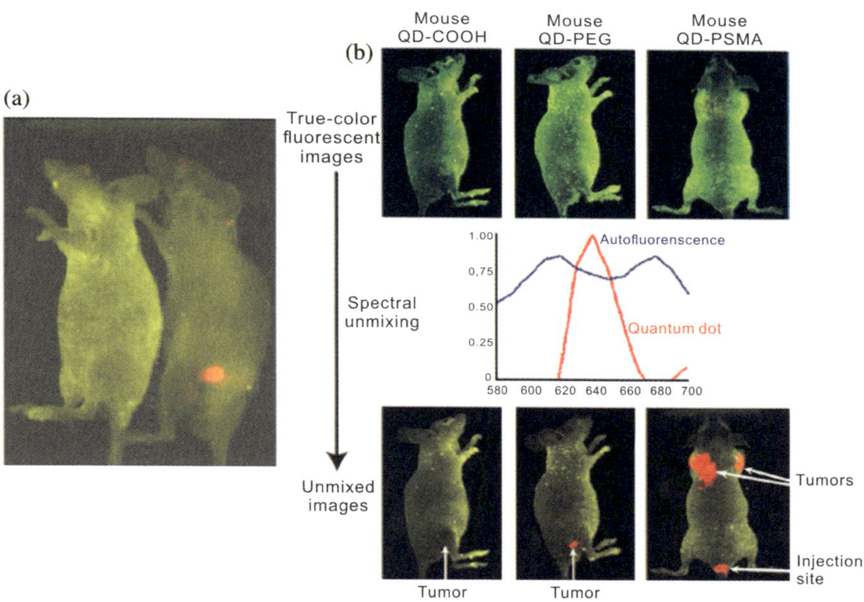

Fig. 2.6. (a) *In vivo* fluorescence of QD-PSMA antibody conjugates in live mice harboring C4-2 tumor xenografts. Orange-red fluorescence signals indicate a prostate tumor growing in a live mouse (right). Control studies using a healthy mouse (no tumor) injected with the same amount of QD probes showed no localized fluorescence signals (left). (b) *In vivo* fluorescence images of tumor-bearing mice using QD probes with three different surface modifications: carboxylic acid groups (left), PEG groups (middle), and PEG-PSMA antibody conjugates (right). Reprinted with permission from Ref. [3]. Copyright (2004) Nature Publishing Group.

antibody, onto the surface of CdSe/ZnS core–shell QDs, and injected these antibody-conjugated QDs (0.4 nmol) into prostate-tumor-bearing mice via tail veins. Subsequent *in vivo* imaging showed that the mouse tumor emitted bright fluorescence after injection (Fig. 2.6a, right). Conversely, no fluorescent spot was observed at the same position as the tumor-bearing mouse for a normal mouse (without a tumor) that was intravenously injected with 0.4 nmol of QD-PSMA antibody (Fig. 2.6a, left). To demonstrate that the active tumor targeting of the QD bioconjugate was much faster and more efficient than the passive targeting of QDs without the tumor-specific ligand, Gao and co-workers injected QD-COOH (6-nmol QDs), QD-PEG (6-nmol QDs) and PEG-QD-PSMA antibody (0.4-nmol QDs) into the tumor-bearing mice. Intense fluorescent signals were observed from mouse tumors only in mice that were injected with the antibody-conjugated QDs. The mice injected with QD-PEG showed weak fluorescence at the tumor site, while those injected with QD-COOH group did not exhibit fluorescent signals from their tumors (Fig. 2.6b). These animal experiments suggest that conjugation of tumor-targeting ligands onto QDs is necessary for *in vivo* solid tumor-targeted imaging because the passive targeting of QDs is much less efficient than active targeting.

Several years later, Papagiannaros *et al.* [15] developed other antibody-coated QD bioprobes for *in vivo* tumor-targeted imaging. They encapsulated NIR QDs into polymeric micelles formed from PEG and phosphatidylethanolamine (PEG-PE) by the thin-layer method, and then conjugated monoclonal antibody 2C5 onto the PEG-PE-coated QDs to form bioprobes with a size of 21.0 ± 6.7 nm. When the QD/(PEG-PE)-2C5 fluorescent bioprobes were injected into the tail veins of mice bearing tumors grown from 4T1 murine breast cancer cells, strong fluorescence was visible from the tumor area 1 h after injection along with autofluorescence from the unmoved hairs. In addition, the average fluorescence intensity of the tumors of mice injected with QD/(PEG-PE)-2C5 was about twice that of tumors of mice injected with nontargeted QD/(PEG-PE) micelles 1 h after injection.

4. Peptide- or Other Small Ligand-conjugated QDs for *In Vivo* Tumor-targeted Imaging

Peptides are considerably smaller than antibodies. The smaller size of nanoparticle-peptide bioconjugates than nanoparticle-antibody bioconjugates may facilitate their migration in animal bodies. In 2002, Akerman *et al.* [2] conjugated thiolated PEG and three peptides with the sequences CGFECVRQCPERC (GFE), KDEPQRRSARLSAKPAPPKPEPKPKKAPAKK (F3) and CGNKRTRGC (LyP-1) onto CdSe/ZnS core–shell QDs. These peptides can bind to various specific tumor cells and their vasculature; e.g., LyP-1 binds to MDA-MB-435 breast cancer cells, but not to lung endothelial cells [2, 16–19]. They injected the QD-peptide bioprobes into the tail veins of mice bearing MDA-MB-435 breast carcinoma xenograft tumors to investigate their tumor targeting. Schematic illustrations of the PEG-conjugated QD-peptides and their tumor targeting are depicted in Fig. 2.7. Microscopic fluorescence imaging of tumor tissue sections showed that QD-F3 and QD-LyP-1 targeted distinct structures within the tumors, In contrast, QD-GFE did not accumulate in the tumors because the breast cancer cells did not express the receptor for the GFE peptide. This is the first example of QD-peptide fluorescent probes that can specifically bind to tumor tissue.

Arginine-glycine-aspartic acid (RGD) peptide is usually used to label nanoparticles for *in vivo* cancer target delivery and imaging. RGD peptide

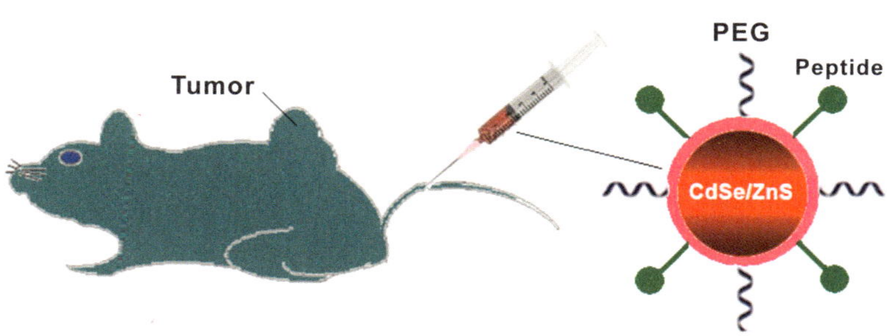

Fig. 2.7. Schematic representation of the intravenous delivery of PEG-conjugated QD-peptides to specific tumor in a mouse.

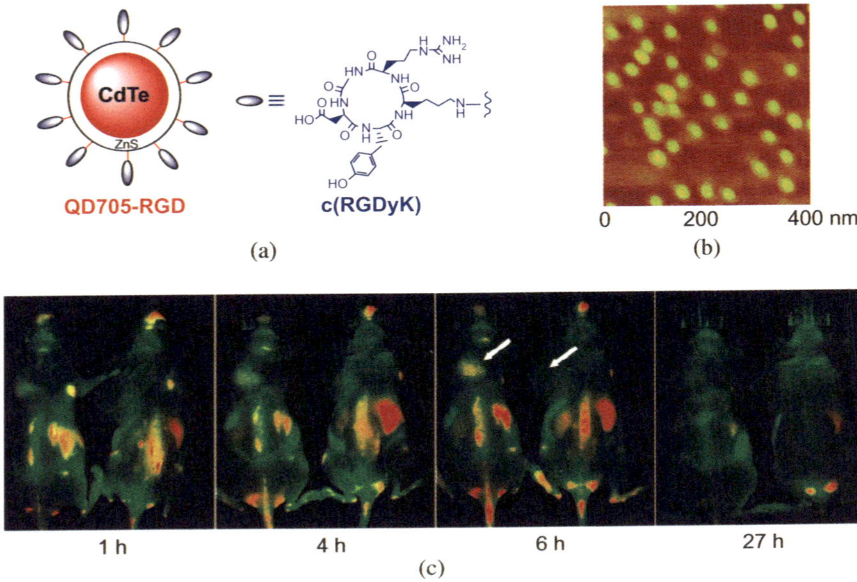

Fig. 2.8. (a) Schematic representations of QD705-RGD (left) and a cyclic RGD molecule (right). (b) Atomic force microscopy (AFM) image of the QD705-RGD. (c) *In vivo* tumor-targeted imaging using QD705-RGD and control QD705. The tail veins of U87MG tumor-bearing mice were injected with 200 pmol of QD705-RGD (left) and QD705 (right). Reprinted with permission from Ref. [20]. Copyright (2006) American Chemical Society.

specifically binds to integrin $\alpha_v\beta_3$-positive tumor vasculature. Because many cancer cells overexpress integrin $\alpha_v\beta_3$ but normal cells do not, RGD-conjugated imaging reagents can therefore be used as diagnostic probes of overexpressed $\alpha_v\beta_3$. In early 2006, Cai *et al.* [20] linked cyclic RGD to QDs with an emission maximum at 705 nm (QD705), as shown in Fig. 2.8a. Both *in vitro* and *ex vivo* experiments demonstrated that the QD705-RGD conjugates with a diameter of 15–20 nm (Fig. 2.8b) could specifically target integrin $\alpha_v\beta_3$. After 200 pmol of QD705-RGD conjugate was intravenously injected into a mouse with an U87MG tumor (human glioblastoma, high integrin $\alpha_v\beta_3$ expression), the fluorescence signal increased over time and reached its maximum 6 h post-injection (Fig. 2.8c, left mouse in each image). However, when the tumor-bearing mouse was injected with 200 pmol of QD705 without conjugated peptide, nearly no marked fluorescence was observed from the tumor site (Fig. 2.8c, right mouse in each image). This may be the first report that RGD peptide-labeled NIR QDs can be used for tumor-targeted imaging in living mice through the specific recognition of integrin $\alpha_v\beta_3$ by QD-RGD. The results show that this technique may provide a novel strategy for cancer diagnosis and imaging-guided management.

During the years following 2006, several further reports showed that QD-RGD bioprobes have great potential for cancer targeted imaging. Coating the QDs with phospholipid vesicles lowers their toxicity and improves their dispersion in aqueous solution. Therefore, the QD surface is usually modified with a hydrophilic lipid shell before bioconjugation (The lipid-coated QDs have been mentioned in the Section 2.2). For example, Yong and co-workers used PEGylated phospholipid micelles to encapsulate NIR CdTe/CdS [5] and CdTe/ZnSe QDs [6], respectively. Cyclic RGD peptide was then conjugated onto the phospholipid micelle-encapsulated QDs. The resulting fluorescent probes CdTe/ZnSe/lipid-RGD and CdTe/CdS/lipid-RGD both exhibited strong capability for *in vivo* tumor targeting and imaging. A pancreatic cancer tumor grown from Panc-1 cells in a mouse intravenously injected with CdTe/ZnSe/lipid-RGD emitted strong NIR fluorescence. Conversely, no obvious NIR fluorescence was detected from the tumor of a mouse treated with unconjugated QDs. In addition, the NIR fluorescent intensity from the tumor site of the CdTe/ZnSe/lipid-RGD-treated mouse was approximately 20- to 25-fold greater than the background autofluorescence 2 h post-injection. These results further indicate that QD-RGD probes can be used specifically for imaging solid tumors including pancreatic cancer tumors.

Because the expression of receptors for folic acid (FA) is upregulated in many human tumors, FA is also commonly conjugated onto the nanoparticles to improve target delivery. For example, Deng *et al.* [7] encapsulated $CuInS_2$/ZnS QDs in FA-modified *N*-succinyl-*N′*-octyl-chitosan micelles to obtain QD/micelle-FA (Fig. 2.9a). The encapsulated QDs were then intravenously injected into mice bearing hepatoma grown from Bel-7402 cancer cells and lung carcinoma grown from A549 cancer cells at a dose of ~8-μg/g body weight. The FA receptor-positive Bel-7402 tumor-bearing mouse emitted bright fluorescence from the tumor tissue 4 h post-injection

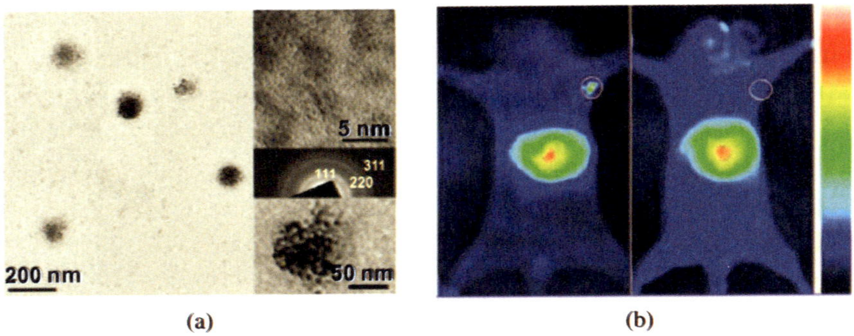

Fig. 2.9. (a) Typical TEM image of $CuInS_2$/ZnS QD-loaded micelles. The insets are a high-resolution TEM image (top) and corresponding selected-area electron diffraction pattern (middle) of the $CuInS_2$/ZnS QDs encapsulated in micelles, and a TEM image of a single QD/micelle nanocomposite (bottom). (b) *In vivo* tumor-targeted imaging using the QD/micelle-FA (left: Bel-7402 tumor-bearing mouse 4 h post-injection, right: A549 tumor-bearing mouse at 4 h post-injection). The tumor site is indicated by a white circle. Reprinted with permission from Ref. [7]. Copyright (2012) American Chemical Society.

(Fig. 2.9b, left). Meanwhile, no obvious fluorescence was observed from the control FA receptor-negative A549 tumor of a mouse 4 h post-injection (Fig. 2.9b, right). The *in vivo* tumor-targeting ability of QD-FA may be similar to that of QD-RGD described above. However, whether the tumor-targeting efficiency of QDs modified with antibody is higher than that of QDs modified with peptide has not yet been systematically studied.

5. Bacteria-coated QDs for *In Vivo* Tumor-targeted Imaging

Typical nanoparticles, including QDs, used for *in vivo* targeted delivery cannot actively recognize the tumor tissue or grow and reproduce in the tumor. However, certain living cells and bacteria tend to actively migrate into tumor tissue and then selectively germinate and grow in it. Bacteria-mediated *in vivo* drug or gene targeted delivery has been investigated for many years using bacteria including *Shigella flexneri*, *Listeria monocytogenes*, *Lactococcus lactis*, *Clostridium novyi-NT*, *Salmonella typhimurium VNP20009*, *Escherichia coli Nissle 1917*, and *bifidobacteria* [21–26].

Bacteria can also be used as a carrier for targeted QD delivery and cancer targeted imaging. In 2012, Liu *et al.* [27] used *Bifidobacterium bifidum* (*B. bifidum*) as a delivery vesicle for CdSeS QDs to allow *in vivo* targeted imaging of solid tumors (lung cancer). *B. bifidum* is a kind of anaerobic bacteria. The oxygen partial pressure in tumor tissue is lower than that in normal tissue [28]. As a result, *B. bifidum* can live between the hypoxic tumor cells, and can also genetically localize and distribute in tumor tissues after intravenous injection [29]. In addition, *B. bifidum* is a probiotic bacteria that is nonpathogenic and nearly nontoxic to the host [21, 30]. Therefore, this type of bacteria has great potential for use in clinical cancer diagnosis and targeted therapy. To reduce the toxicity of the QDs to *B. bifidum* and increase the QD loading capacity, Liu *et al.* [27] encapsulated the QDs in palmitoyloleoylphosphatidylcholine (POPC) micelles and then accelerated the migration of QDs into the bacteria using an electroporation technique. The surface of the QD-loaded bacteria was further conjugated with FA to improve the specificity of *in vivo* tumor targeting by the bacteria. Schematic illustrations of the formation of QD/bacteria-FA bioconjugates and their administration are depicted in Fig. 2.10. Because the permeability of the cell plasma membrane would be obviously increased by externally applied electroporation, most of the bacteria (>66.8%) were loaded with the POPC-coated QDs after the bacteria were stimulated by the electrical field under the optimum experimental conditions (Fig. 2.11a). After the QD/bacteria-FA bioconjugates

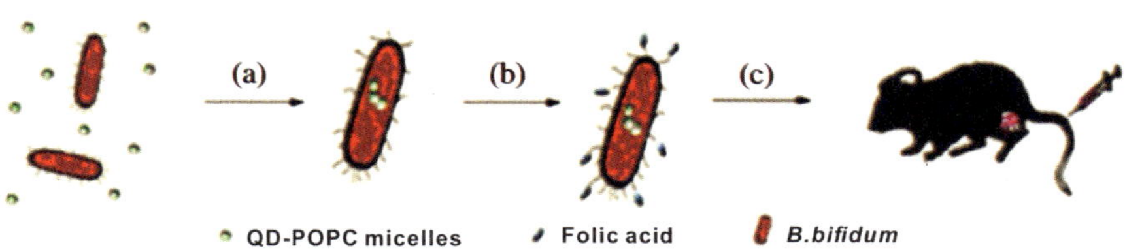

Fig. 2.10. Schematic illustrations of QD loading and *in vivo* tumor imaging. (a) Loading *B. bifidum* with QDs via electroporation, (b) surface modification of *B. bifidum* with FA, and (c) intravenous administration of the bioconjugate. Reprinted with permission from Ref. [27]. Copyright (2012) Elsevier.

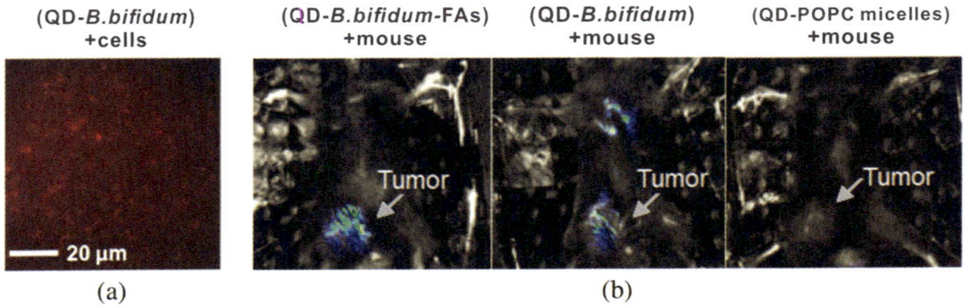

Fig. 2.11. (a) Fluorescence image of QD-bacteria bioconjugate, and (b) for *in vivo* tumor-targeted imaging using the QD-bacteria-FA bioconjugate. Reprinted with permission from Ref. [27]. Copyright (2012) Elsevier.

(200 μL, 1×10^5/mL for each mouse) were intravenously injected into tumor-bearing mouse, the tumor site emitted bright fluorescence (Fig. 2.11b, left). When the QD/bacteria composite without FA was injected into a tumor-bearing mouse, the QD/bacteria composite accumulated not only in the tumor tissue but also in other organs such as lungs (Fig. 2.11b, middle). Meanwhile, when a tumor-bearing mouse was injected with POPC-coated QDs alone (without bacteria and FA), no obvious fluorescence was detected because the QDs were dispersed throughout its body (Fig. 2.11b, right). This study indicates that ligand-conjugated probiotic bacteria may be suitable as QD carriers for *in vivo* cancer detection.

6. Trajectory of Targeted Delivery of a Single QD Bioconjugate to Tumor Cells in Live Mice

The targeted delivery of QD bioconjugates to tumor tissue *in vivo* after intravenous injection is a complex process. In 2007, Tada *et al.* [31] tracked a single QD-trastuzumab bioconjugate nanoparticle in nude BALB/c mice bearing KPL-4 breast cancer xenograft tumors using a dorsal skinfold chamber and a high-speed confocal microscope equipped with a high-sensitivity camera. Trastuzumab (trade name Herceptin) is a humanized anti-Her2 receptor monoclonal antibody that is mainly used clinically to treat certain breast cancers. Tada *et al.* [31] conjugated NIR QDs with an emission wavelength of 800 nm with trastuzumab and then injected the resulting QD-trastuzumab bioconjugate (2 μmol/L, 100 μL) into the tail vein of mice with HER2-overexpressing breast cancer. They found that the current of the QD-trastuzumab bioconjugates in a tumor vessel could be observed within 30 s after injection, and the average movement speed of each QD-trastuzumab bioconjugate in the bloodstream ranged from 100 to 600 μm/s. By 2 h post-injection, many bioconjugates had migrated into the tumor interstitial area close to the tumor vessels with an average diffusion coefficient of 0.0014 μm^2/s. At 6 h post-injection, the bioconjugates had moved from the interstitial space near the tumor vessels toward the cancer cell membrane at a speed of 200 to 400 nm/s. The bioconjugates then bound to HER2 protein on the breast cancer cell membrane. In a given cell, the bioconjugates changed direction so they were parallel to the cell membrane, migrated into the intracellular space and then moved toward the cell nucleus at a higher speed of ~600 nm/s. In addition, the bioconjugates near the nucleus moved within a small area with random orientation and speed; the directional movement ceased. Of course, the rate of movement of the nanoparticles in each of the above processes is influenced by many factors such as the size and Zeta potential of the nanoparticles. Tada and co-workers concluded that the transport trajectory of the QD-trastuzumab bioconjugate after injection involved six stages: vessel circulation, extravasation, movement into the extracellular region, binding to HER2 on the cell membrane, movement from the cell membrane to the perinuclear region after endocytosis, and movement in the perinuclear region.

7. Discussion

In vivo tumor-targeted imaging with QDs has been successfully used in live animals. This technique not only can be used for rapidly detecting the exact location of solid tumors, but also may be used for seeing whether drugs conjugated with QDs can accumulate in tumors without killing the host animals. This direction of biomedical research on QDs has grown rapidly during the past about 15 years. The tumor-targeting efficiency of the QDs is an important factor influencing the sensitivity of detection. The conjugation of biorecognition molecules such as antibodies, peptides and ligands on QD surfaces can facilitate the specific accumulation of QDs in tumor tissue. Antibodies are usually more stable in blood than other small biorecognition molecules such as peptides. However, the molecular weights of most antibodies exceed 100,000. Therefore, the conjugation of such large antibodies to the QDs will markedly increase their hydrodynamic diameter, which increases the steric hindrance to QDs migrating in blood. In addition, large QD bioconjugates cannot easily penetrate into solid tumors. Ligands and peptides are smaller than monoclonal antibodies, such biomolecules may possess higher tumor-targeting specificity. Recombinant antibody fragments may be a good candidate to improve the tumor-targeting efficiency of QDs. This is because antibody fragments are much smaller than whole antibodies but they still retain the tumor-targeting specificity of whole monoclonal antibody [32]. Besides the biorecognition molecules described above, the tumor-targeting efficiency of QDs is also seriously affected by the hydrodynamic diameter and surface charge of the QD composites and their nonspecific uptake by the liver and spleen and other organs.

The toxicity and slow clearance of QDs *in vivo* may be the biggest obstacles that currently prevent the use of QDs in clinical diagnosis. The toxicity of QDs is an intrinsic property. Surface modification of QDs can only decrease their toxicity rather than remove it entirely. It has been demonstrated that QDs with hydrodynamic diameter >15 nm introduced by intravenous injection are difficult to clear from the body through renal excretion; only QDs with hydrodynamic diameter ≤5.5 nm are rapidly eliminated [33]. Therefore, unless ultra-low toxic QDs have been developed, the possibility of clinical translation of *in vivo* tumor-targeted imaging using QDs may be low at present.

References

[1] Han MY, Gao XH, Su JZ and Nie S. (2001). Quantum-dot-tagged microbeads for multiplexed optical coding of biomolecules. *Nat. Biotechnol.*, **19**:631–635.

[2] Akerman ME, Chan WCW, Laakkonen P, Bhatia SN and Ruoslahti E. (2002). Nanocrystal targeting *in vivo*. *PNAS*, **99**:12617–12621.

[3] Gao XH, Cui YY, Levenson RM, Chung LWK and Nie SM. (2004). *In vivo* cancer targeting and imaging with semiconductor quantum dots. *Nat. Biotechnol.*, **22**:969–976.

[4] Yong KT, Hu R, Roy I, Ding H, Vathy LA, Bergey EJ, Mizuma M, Maitra A and Prasad PN. (2009). tumor targeting and imaging in live animals with functionalized semiconductor quantum rods. *ACS Appl. Mat. Interfaces*, **1**:710–719.

[5] Yong KT. (2010). Biophotonics and biotechnology in pancreatic cancer: cyclic RGD-peptide-conjugated type II quantum dots for *in vivo* imaging. *Pancreatology*, **10**:553–564.

[6] Yong KT, Roy I, Law WC and Hu R. (2010). Synthesis of cRGD-peptide conjugated near-infrared CdTe/ZnSe core-shell quantum dots for *in vivo* cancer targeting and imaging. *Chem. Commun.*, **46**:7136–7138.

[7] Deng DW, Chen YQ, Cao J, Tian JM, Qian ZY, Achilefu S and Gu YQ. (2012). High-Quality CuInS2/ZnS Quantum Dots for *in vitro* and *in vivo* Bioimaging. *Chem. Mater.*, **24**:3029–3037.

[8] Shuhendler AJ, Prasad P, Chan HK, Gordijo CR, Soroushian B, Kolios M, Yu K, O'Brien PJ, Rauth AM and Wu XY. (2011). Hybrid quantum dot-fatty ester stealth nanoparticles: toward clinically relevant *in vivo* optical imaging of deep tissue. *Acs Nano.*, **5**:1958–1966.

[9] Hong GS, Robinson JT, Zhang YJ, Diao S, Antaris AL, Wang QB and Dai H. (2012). *In vivo* fluorescence imaging with Ag2S quantum dots in the second near-infrared region. *Angew. Chem. Int. Edit.*, **51**:9818–9821.

[10] Smith AM, Duan HW, Mohs AM and Nie SM. (2008). Bioconjugated quantum dots for *in vivo* molecular and cellular imaging. *Adv Drug Deliv. Rev.*, **60**:1226–1240.

[11] Matsumura Y and Maeda H. (1986). A new concept for macromolecular therapeutics in cancer chemotherapy: mechanism of tumoritropic accumulation of proteins and the antitumor agent smancs. *Cancer Res.*, **46**:6387–6392.

[12] Skinner SA, Tutton PJ and O'Brien PE. (1990). Microvascular architecture of experimental colon tumors in the rat. *Cancer Res.*, **50**:2411–2417.

[13] Iyer AK, Khaled G, Fang J and Maeda H. (2006). *Drug Discov. Today*, **11**:812–818.

[14] Al-Jamal WT, Al-Jamal KT, Tian B, Cakebread A, Halket JM and Kostarelos K. (2009). Tumor targeting of functionalized quantum dot-liposome hybrids by intravenous administration. *Mol. Pharm.*, **6**:520–530.

[15] Papagiannaros A, Upponi J, Hartner W, Mongayt D, Levchenko T and Torchilin V. (2010). Quantum dot loaded immunomicelles for tumor imaging. *BMC Med. Imaging*, **10**:22.

[16] Rajotte D, Arap W, Hagedorn M, Koivunen E, Pasqualini R and Ruoslahti E. (1998). Molecular heterogeneity of the vascular endothelium revealed by *in vivo* phage display. *J. clin. invest.*, **102**:430–437.

[17] Rajotte D and Ruoslahti E. (1999). Membrane dipeptidase is the receptor for a lung-targeting peptide identified by *in vivo* phage display. *J. Biol. Chem.*, **274**:11593–11598.

[18] Porkka K, Laakkonen P, Hoffman JA, Bernasconi M and Ruoslahti E. (2002). A fragment of the HMGN2 protein homes to the nuclei of tumor cells and tumor endothelial cells *in vivo*. *PNAS*, **99**:7444–7449.

[19] Laakkonen P, Porkka K, Hoffman JA and Ruoslahti E. (2002). A tumor-homing peptide with a targeting specificity related to lymphatic vessels. *Nat. Med.*, **8**:751–755.

[20] Cai W, Shin DW, Chen K, Gheysens O, Cao Q, Wang SX, Gambhir SS and Chen X. (2006). Peptide-labeled near-infrared quantum dots for imaging tumor vasculature in living subjects. *Nano Lett.*, **6**:669–676.

[21] Ryan RM, Green J and Lewis CE. (2006). Use of bacteria in anti-cancer therapies. *Bioessays*. **28**:84–94.

[22] Diaz Jr LA, Cheong I, Foss CA, Zhang XS, Peters BA, Agrawal N, Bettegowda C, Karim B, Liu G, Khan K, Huang X, Kohli M, Dang LH, Hwang P, Vogelstein A, Garrett Mayer E, Kobrin B, Pomper M, Zhou S, Kinzler KW, Vogelstein B and Huso DL. (2005). Pharmacologic and toxicologic evaluation of C-novyi-NT spores. *Toxicol. Sci.*, **88**:562–575.

[23] Jia LJ, Xu HM, Ma DY, Hu QG, Huang XF, Jiang WH, Li SF, Jia KZ, Huang QL and Hua ZC. (2005). Enhanced therapeutic effect by combination of tumor-targeting Salmonella and endostatin in murine melanoma model. *Cancer Biol. Ther.*, **4**:840–845.

[24] Stritzker J, Weibel S, Hill PJ, Oelschlaeger TA, Goebel W and Szalay AA. (2007). Tumor-specific colonization, tissue distribution, and gene induction by probiotic Escherichia coli Nissle 1917 in live mice. *Int. J. Med. Microbiol.*, **297**:151–162.

[25] Li X, Fu GF, Fan YR, Liu WH, Liu XJ, Wang JJ and Xu GX. (2003). Bifidobacterium adolescentis as a delivery system of endostatin for cancer

gene therapy: Selective inhibitor of angiogenesis and hypoxic tumor growth. *Cancer Gene. Ther.*, **10**:105–111.

[26] Yazawa K, Fujimori M, Nakamura T, Sasaki T, Amano J, Kano Y and Taniguchi S. (2001). Bifidobacterium longum as a delivery system for gene therapy of chemically induced rat mammary tumors. *Breast Cancer Res. Tr.*, **66**:165–170.

[27] Liu Y, Zhou M, Luo D, Wang LJ, Hong YK, Yang YP and Sha YL. (2012). Bacteria-mediated *in vivo* delivery of quantum dots into solid tumor. *Biochem. Biophys. Res. Commun.*, **425**:769–774.

[28] Vaupel PW. (1993). Oxygenation of solid tumors in drug resistance in oncology. In: Teicher BA, ed. New York: Marcel Dekker; 53–85.

[29] Yazawa K, Fujimori M, Amano J, Kano Y and Taniguchi S. (2000). Bifidobacterium longum as a delivery system for cancer gene therapy: Selective localization and growth in hypoxic tumors. *Cancer Gene. Ther.*, **7**:269–274.

[30] Dang LH, Bettegowda C, Huso DL, Kinzler KW and Vogelstein B. (2001). Combination bacteriolytic therapy for the treatment of experimental tumors. *PNAS*, **98**:15155–15160.

[31] Tada H, Higuchi H, Wanatabe TM and Ohuchi N. (2007). *In vivo* real-time tracking of single quantum dots conjugated with monoclonal anti-HER2 antibody in tumors of mice. *Cancer Res.*, **67**:1138–1144.

[32] Holliger P and Hudson PJ. (2005). Engineered antibody fragments and the rise of single domains. *Nat. Biotechnol.*, **23**:1126–1136.

[33] Choi HS, Liu W, Misra P, Tanaka E, Zimmer JP, Ipe BI, Bawendi MG and Frangioni JV. (2007). Renal clearance of quantum dots. *Nat. Biotechnol.*, **25**:1165–1170.

Chapter 3

Self-Illuminating Quantum Dots for *In Vivo* Imaging

In vivo near-infrared (NIR) fluorescent imaging has several advantages, such as good biological safety (e.g., no radiological hazard), quantitative sensitivity, easy operation, and real-time imaging. However, this noninvasive imaging technique is difficult to use for deep tissue detection because the ability of NIR light to penetrate animal tissues is limited, and animal tissues also usually have strong background autofluorescence. These limitations can be overcome by optical imaging based on bioluminescence resonance energy transfer (BRET). In this chapter, red and NIR semiconductor quantum dot (QD)-BRET systems and their use *in vivo* imaging in small animals are discussed. In the QD-BRET systems considered here, red or NIR QDs are conjugated with an eight-mutation variant of *Rotylenchulus reniformis* luciferase (Luc8). When the QD-Luc8 bioconjugates encounter the substrate coelenterazine, Luc8 emits blue luminescence and this light energy is transferred from Luc8 to the QDs. This allows the QDs to emit red or NIR fluorescence without external excitation. This bioluminescence imaging technique can be used for deep tissue detection without interference from tissue autofluorescence, which is interesting to both materials and biomedical scientists.

1. Introduction

Clinical diagnosis using imaging techniques such as magnetic resonance, computed tomography, ultrasonic, and X-ray imaging can rapidly reveal the position and shape of local lesions in deep tissue. *In vivo* near-infrared (NIR) fluorescence imaging is a novel technique developed in the last about 15 years. Advantages of NIR fluorescence imaging include quantitative sensitivity, inherent biological safety, relative ease of use [1], and real-time imaging. This noninvasive imaging technique has been used in small-animal research. However, compared with the traditional imaging methods noted above, current fluorescence imaging techniques are not suitable for clinical diagnosis of local lesions in deep tissue.

Chapters 1 and 2 described *in vivo* imaging using QDs, which is a type of fluorescence imaging. Although the NIR fluorescence of QDs can penetrate animal tissue, external excitation light needs to be applied to induce emission from the QDs trapped in tissue. This process is limited by the strong background autofluorescence from ubiquitous endogenous chromophores, and the absorption and scattering of optical photons in tissues. As a result, QDs trapped in deep tissue only receive a small proportion of external excitation light [2], and only a part of the QD fluorescence can be detected outside the body.

These limitations may be overcome by bioluminescence imaging. Bioluminescence imaging is an optical detection technique where visible light is produced by a chemical reaction between enzyme and substrate in a living organism. Bioluminescence can penetrate several centimeters of tissue [3]. When QDs are combined with a bioluminescent material to form a system that operates based on BRET, the sensitivity of *in vivo* imaging using QDs can be greatly improved compared with that of fluorescence imaging with QDs alone.

2. BRET and QDs as an Energy Acceptor in BRET

BRET is a nonradiative process where the energy generated by a suitable donor (e.g., luciferase) is transferred to an acceptor (e.g., fluorescent protein) based on the Förster mechanism. To obtain efficient BRET, the fluorescent emission spectrum of the donor should overlap with the excitation spectrum of the acceptor, and the distance between donor and acceptor moieties must be less than about 10 nm [4]. In BRET, external excitation light is not required because the energy used to excite the acceptor is bioluminescence generated by a chemical reaction between a luciferase and a substrate. Therefore, *in vivo* imaging with a BRET system is more sensitive than *in vivo* fluorescence imaging because background interference and tissue attenuation associated with excitation and emission light are minimized.

BRET donors include renilla luciferase (Rluc), aequorin and firefly luciferase, and the acceptors include fluorescent proteins, small organic dyes and fluorescent nanoparticles like QDs (Fig. 3.1) [5]. Compared with

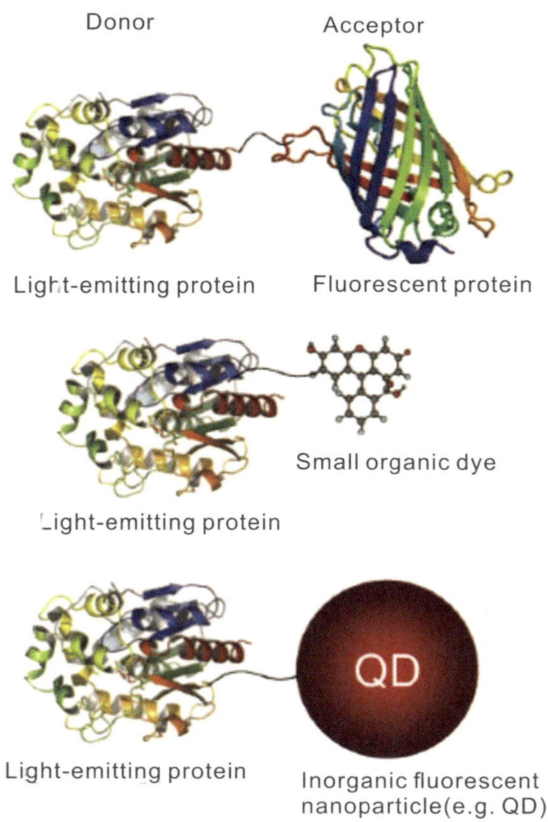

Fig. 3.1. BRET can occur between a light-emitting protein (donor) and different fluorophores (acceptors). Reprinted with permission from Ref. [5]. Copyright (2009) Elsevier.

fluorescent proteins and small-molecule fluorophores, QDs as BRET acceptors have a large Stokes shift (large gap between the emission peaks of the donor and acceptor) because QDs have narrow emission bandwidths [5]. In addition, QDs have broad continuous absorption spectra ranging from ultraviolet to visible regions, which allow them to be conveniently excited by different wavelengths. Also, QDs can be modulated to emit red or NIR fluorescence by controlling their particle size, which can overcome the obstacle faced by fluorescent proteins of only emitting at short wavelengths [5].

BRET has mainly been used for the detection of nucleic acid targets, protein–protein or protein–ligand interactions, and *in vivo* imaging. For example, Fig. 3.2 shows a BRET-based nucleic acid sensing system [6]. In this sensing platform, two small antisense oligonucleotide sequences are covalently attached to Rluc or a semiconductor QD. Rluc, which generates light by a chemical reaction, is used as an energy donor to provide an excitation source for the QD, while the QD acts as an energy acceptor and then emits fluorescence. The Rluc- and QD-labeled sequences hybridize to the target in a head-to-head fashion. Energy is then transferred from Rluc to the QD upon addition of the substrate coelenterazine, leading to fluorescence emission from the QD. This BRET-based sensing system

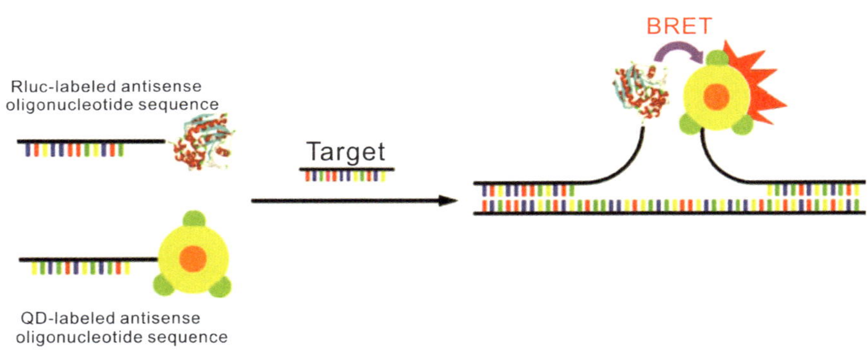

Fig. 3.2. Schematic diagram of a BRET-based on-type nucleic acid sensing system. Reprinted with permission from Ref. [6]. Copyright (2011) Elsevier.

containing Rluc and QDs can detect target nucleic acids in buffer as well as in the cellular matrix of *Escherichia coli* with high sensitivity.

Another example is red light-emitting BRET systems that have been developed for *in vitro* and *in vivo* analysis of protein–protein interactions. The drug rapamycin can efficiently induce a molecular interaction between 12-kDa immunosuppressant drug FK506 binding protein (FKBP12) and FKBP12 rapamycin binding domain (FRB) [7]. This drug-induced molecular interaction has been widely used for protein–protein interaction assays. In 2011, Dragulescu-Andrasi *et al.* [8] conjugated FRB onto Rluc8.6 as an energy donor, and red fluorescent protein TurboFP635 as an energy acceptor onto FKBP12. When coelenterazine and rapamycin were added to this system, the rapamycin-induced interaction of FRB and FKBP12 juxtaposed FRB-Rluc8.6 and FKBP12-TurboFP635. As a result, TurboFP635 was excited by the bioluminescence generated by the reaction between Rluc8.6 and luciferase substrate coelenterazine. Finally, the red fluorescence from TurboFP635 was detected. The bioluminescence of Rluc8.6 and fluorescence of TurboFP635 appear at 535 and 635 nm, respectively, so the difference between these two emission peaks is 100 nm. This BRET system is suitable for analysis of protein–protein interactions in living animals. HT1080 cells expressing FRB-Rluc8.6 and FKBP12-TurboFP635 were injected into the tail vein of mice. Two hours later, rapamycin and coelenterazine dissolved in dimethyl sulfoxide (DMSO) were intravenously injected into the same mice, resulting in bright luminescence from the mouse lungs compared with that from the control group. This is because FRB-Rluc8.6 and FKBP12-TurboFP635 were trapped in the lungs after injection and then formed FRB-Rluc8.6/FKBP12-TurboFP635 pairs in the presence of rapamycin. The luminescence observed from the lungs was the fluorescence of TurboFP635 generated by BRET between Rluc8.6 and TurboFP635.

3. Self-Illuminating QDs

Light-emitting protein-conjugated QD systems that operate through the efficient transfer of bioluminescence energy from a protein to a QD to

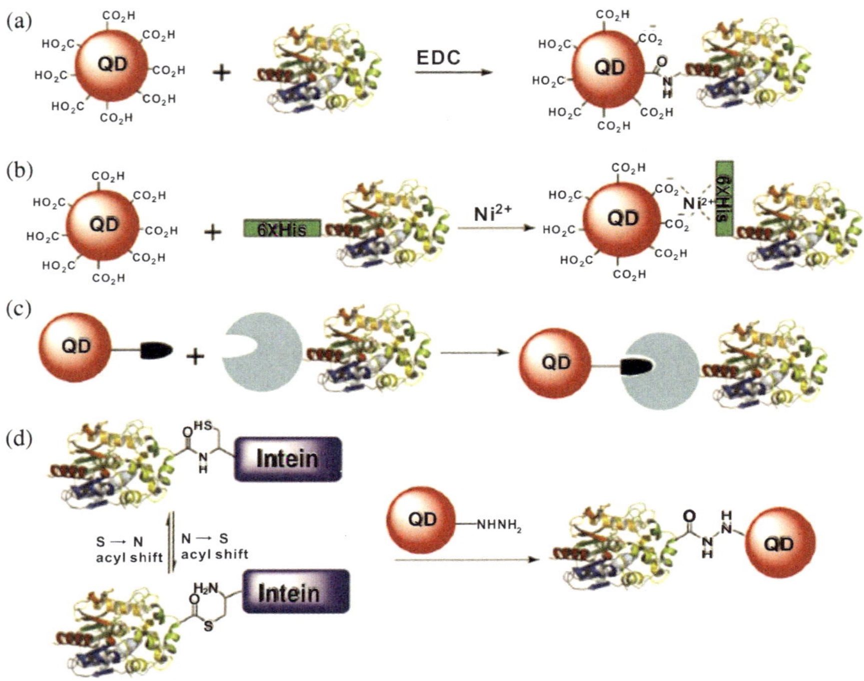

Fig. 3.3. Four approaches used to conjugate light-emitting proteins to QDs. (a) EDC-mediated conjugation of bioluminescent protein Luc8 to carboxylate-coated QDs. (b) Metal ion (Ni^{2+})-mediated complexation of QDs and Luc8. (c) Specific interaction mediated by protein–ligand interactions. (d) Intein-mediated site-specific conjugation of Luc8 to QDs. Reprinted with permission from Ref. [5]. Copyright (2009) Elsevier.

induce QD emission are named self-illuminating QDs. The conjugation of the light-emitting protein to the QD surface is an important step to generate self-illuminating QDs with highly efficient BRET. Rao and colleagues have summarized the four current approaches to obtain QD-BRET systems, which are presented in Fig. 3.3 [5]. The first method is based on amide formation through reaction of amine and carboxyl groups mediated by 1-ethyl-3-(3-dimethylaminopropyl) carbodiimide hydrochloride (EDC), which has been widely used to prepare QD bio-conjugates. Generally, QD surfaces are modified with carboxylate groups, which then react with amino groups on the light-emitting protein (e.g., luciferase) to form amide-linked composites (Fig. 3.3a). The second is metal-mediated complexation between the light-emitting protein and QDs (Fig. 3.3b). For example, a short peptide of 15 amino acids containing matrix metalloproteinase and six-histidine tag (6xHis) was genetically fused to the eight-mutation variant of *Rotylenchulus reniformis* luciferase (Luc8) [9]. After Ni^{2+} cations were mixed with carboxyl-modified QDs, the carboxylic acid moieties bound to the Ni^{2+} ions to form complexes with the 6xHis on Luc8 to give a self-illuminating Luc8-6xHis-QD conjugate. The third method to form QD-BRET systems is based on protein–protein or protein–ligand interactions (Fig. 3.3c), which was discussed above in Fig. 3.2. The fourth approach is the intein-mediated direct site-specific conjugation of a light-emitting protein to QDs (Fig. 3.3d) [10].

In 2006, Rao *et al.* [2] first used bioluminescence from a protein to excite QDs and develop self-illuminating QDs. They conjugated Luc8 onto polymer-coated CdSe/ZnS core–shell QDs with an emission wavelength of 655 nm [QD(655)] via amide formation in the presence of the coupling reagent EDC. After addition of the substrate coelenterazine, Luc8 emitted blue luminescence, which was then transferred from Luc8 to the QDs to trigger red fluorescence from the QDs provided the distance between the Luc8 shell and QD core was less than ~10 nm (Fig. 3.4a). Compared with other light-emitting proteins, Luc8 exhibits high stability in biological media, and its bioluminescence overlaps well with the absorption spectrum of QD(655), which is required for efficient energy transfer. As a result, the QD(655)-Luc8 conjugate exhibited highly efficient BRET. As shown in Fig. 3.4b, when coelenterazine was added to QD(655)-Luc8 conjugate, two emission peaks were observed: the bioluminescence of Luc8 at 480 nm, and the strong fluorescence emission from QD(655) at 655 nm. The difference between these two emission peaks is 175 nm. The efficiency of BRET in the QD(655)-Luc8 system was 56%.

Because the fluorescence of semiconductor QDs can be modulated by changing their size, self-illuminating QDs with numerous luminescence emission peaks may be conveniently prepared. For example, when Luc8

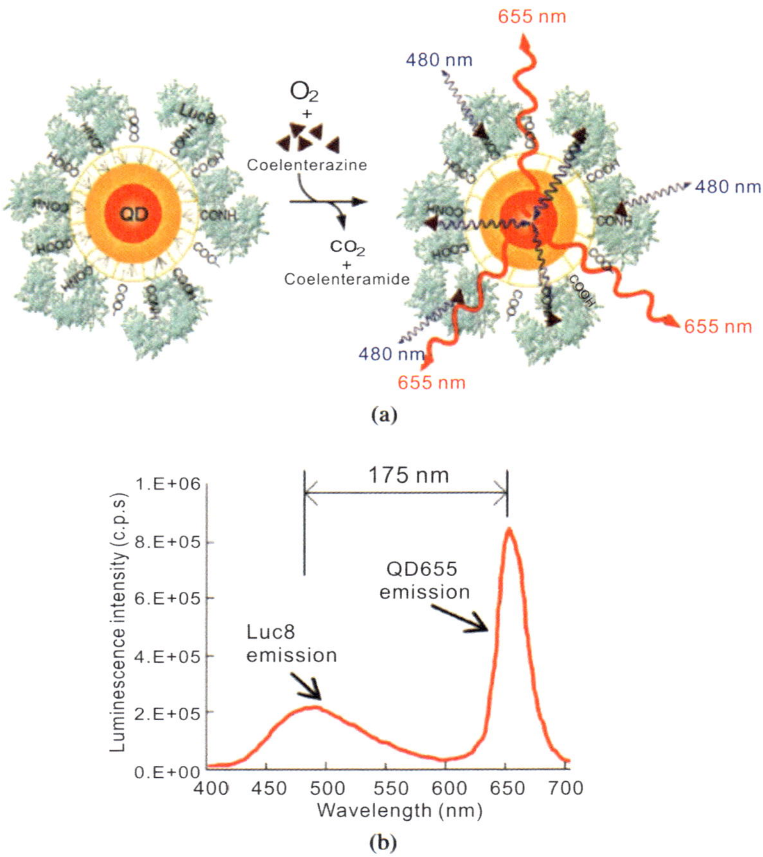

Fig. 3.4. (a) Schematic illustration of a self-illuminating QD and the mechanism of BRET between QD(655) and Luc8. (b) Emission spectrum of QD(655)-Luc8 showing BRET from Luc8 to QD(655). Reprinted with permission from Ref. [2]. Copyright (2006) Nature Publishing Group.

was covalently conjugated onto QDs with emission wavelengths of 605, 655, 705, and 800 nm [named QD(605), QD(655), QD(705) and QD(800), respectively], four separated fluorescence emissions at wavelengths longer than 600 nm could be simultaneously detected after the addition of coelenterazine (Fig. 3.5) [5], indicating that BRET occurred in all four of the QD-Luc8 conjugates.

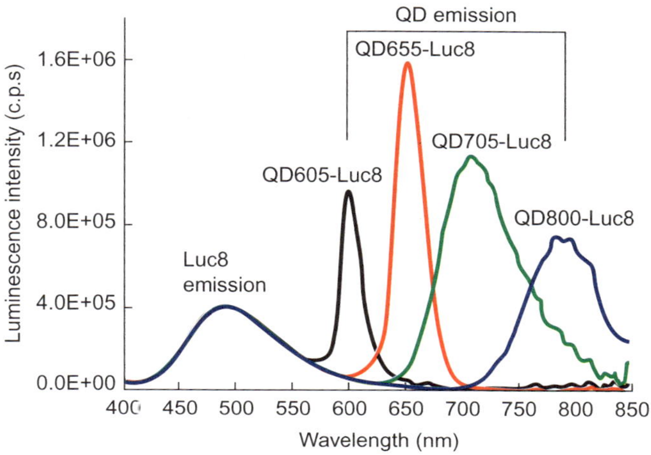

Fig. 3.5. Emission spectra of four self-illuminating QDs (QD(605)-Luc8, QD(655)-Luc8, QD(705)-Luc8, and QD(800)-Luc8) based on BRET. Reprinted with permission from Ref. [5]. Copyright (2009) Elsevier.

4. Sensitivity of *In Vivo* Optical Imaging Using Self-illuminating QDs

Rao and co-workers [2] first demonstrated that self-illuminating QDs could be used for *in vivo* deep tissue detection with no background interference. They conjugated a polycationic peptide (arginine 9-mer, denoted hereafter as R9) onto the QD(655)-Luc8 bioconjugates described above to improve their cellular uptake efficiency. The resulting QD(655)-Luc8-R9 nanoconjugate was incubated with C6 rat glioma cells for 1 h. As shown in Fig. 3.6a, each cell emitted bright fluorescence. To investigate whether the QD(655)-Luc8-R9 nanoconjugate in living cells could undergo BRET after the addition of coelenterazine, the QD(655)-Luc8-R9 nanoconjugate-labeled cells were collected by trypsinization or cell scraping, incubated with coelenterazine, and then imaged by a bioluminescence imaging method. The results showed that QD(655)-Luc8-R9 in cells emitted bright fluorescence (BRET filter: 575–650 nm) without external excitation (Fig. 3.6b, left tube), indicating that BRET occurred

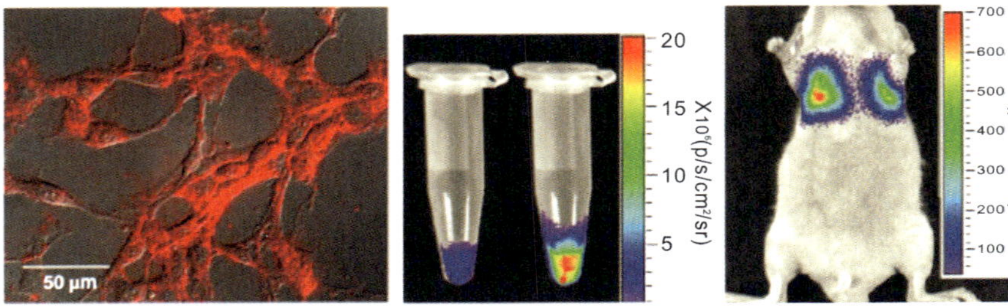

Fig. 3.6. (a) Fluorescence image of C6 rat glioma cells labeled with QD(655)-Luc8-R9. (b) Coelenterazine was added to the QD(655)-Luc8-R9-labeled cells and imaged by *in vivo* bioluminescence imaging. Left tube: acquired with a filter (575–650 nm); Right tube: no filter. (c) Nude mouse injected with the QD(655)-Luc8-R9-labeled cells via the tail vein and imaged with *in vivo* bioluminescence imaging (no filter). Reprinted with permission from Ref. [2]. Copyright (2006) Nature Publishing Group.

after QD(655)-Luc8-R9 was taken into the cells. If the bioluminescence of Luc8 was not filtered, the emission intensity of QD(655)-Luc8-R9 in the cells (Fig. 3.6b, right tube) was about five times higher than that of the sample in the left tube. They then intravenously injected the QD(655)-Luc8-R9-labeled cells (~2×10^6) and coelenterazine (10 μg) into a mouse. The cells accumulated in the lungs of the mouse, which was observed clearly by the BRET signal, and no background light was observed from the other parts of the mouse (Fig. 3.6c). In addition, compared with the results of *in vivo* bioluminescence imaging, the fluorescence signal from the mouse lungs was difficult to observe when the mouse was imaged with *in vivo* fluorescence imaging. This suggests that *in vivo* bioluminescence imaging with self-illuminating QDs is superior to *in vivo* fluorescence imaging with QDs.

Self-illuminating QDs with different fluorescence emission peaks may be simultaneously used for *in vivo* bioluminescence imaging based on BRET. For example, when a mouse was injected with C6 glioma cells labeled with QD(655)-Luc8 and QD(800)-Luc8 in the tail and intramuscularly, respectively, followed by injection with coelenterazine and imaging, both conjugates could be simultaneously imaged without external excitation, and their emission could be identified by using emission filters with different wavelengths [2].

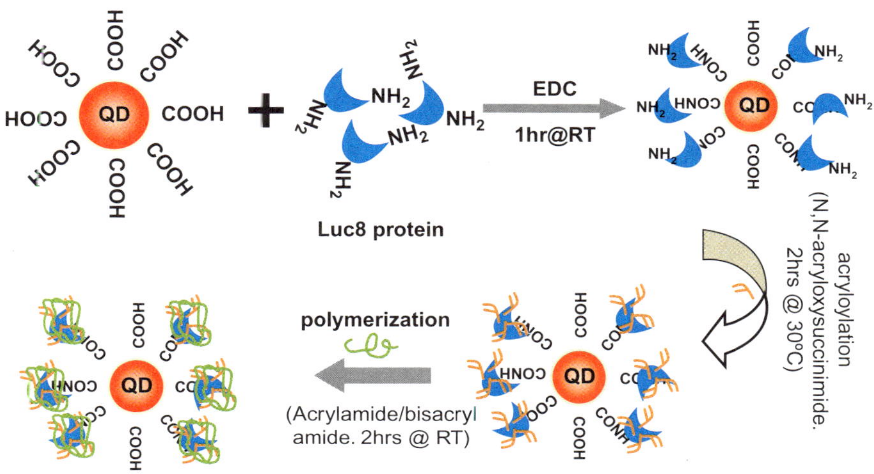

Fig. 3.7. Schematic illustration of the formation of a QD-Luc8 bioconjugate and its subsequent encapsulation. Reprinted with permission from Ref. [11]. Copyright (2008) Elsevier.

However, the emission stability of QD-Luc8 bioconjugates in blood or serum is limited, which is a disadvantage for long-term *in vivo* imaging. In 2008, Rao and colleagues developed a technique to improve the stability of the Luc8 enzyme on QDs [11]. They incubated QD(655)-Luc8 conjugates with acrylic acid N-hydroxysuccinimide ester to generate surface vinyl groups, and then encapsulated the Luc8 proteins by *in situ* polymerization at room temperature using acrylamide as the monomer (Fig. 3.7). The resulting polymer-encapsulated QD(655)-Luc8 conjugates remained fairly stable in serum at 37°C for up to 5 days (37% bioluminescence retained) and in phosphate buffer at 4°C for over 4 months (more than 30% activity retained). In contrast, the unencapsulated QD(655)-Luc8 conjugates retained only around 5–10% of their initial bioluminescence after 48 h in mouse serum at 37°C. Similar interesting findings were found in animal experiments. Polymer-encapsulated QD(655)-Luc8 and unmodified QD(655)-Luc8 conjugates containing 5 pmol of QDs were subcutaneously injected into mice, and after 2 min, coelenterazine was injected into the mice via the tail vein. As shown in Fig. 3.8, the bioluminescence of the encapsulated conjugates (left side) was much more stable than that of the unmodified conjugates (right side), with or without a BRET filter.

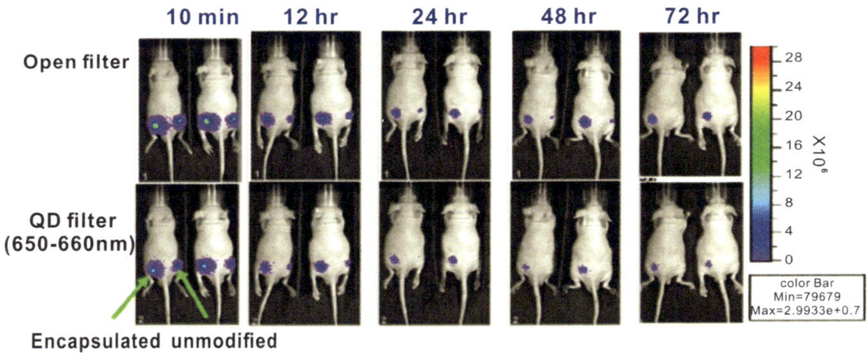

Fig. 3.8. *In vivo* luminescence stability of polymer-encapsulated and unmodified QD(655)-Luc8. Both types of self-illuminating QDs were injected subcutaneously into the left or right side of the same mouse followed by intravenous injection of coelenterazine and bioluminescence imaging. Because QD filter only collected light emitting between 650 and 660 nm, the emission observed from the mouse is mainly QD fluorescence generated by BRET. Reprinted with permission from Ref. [11]. Copyright (2008) Elsevier.

In 2012, our research group [12] prepared self-illuminating QDs using cadmium telluride (CdTe)/cadmium sulfide (CdS) QDs as the energy acceptor of BRET and Luc8 as the energy donor. Both the CdTe/CdS QDs and QD-Luc8 bioconjugate emitted bright fluorescence after being excited at 630 nm. When the QD-Luc8 bioconjugate encountered coelenterazine, Luc8 and coelenterazine reacted to generate blue light of ~480 nm, and this light excited the QDs to emit red fluorescence. To compare the depth of tissue penetration achievable by the emission of the CdTe/CdS QDs, Luc8 and QD-Luc8, we used a series of hairless pig skins with different thicknesses to cover the three samples. The luminescence of the QD-Luc8 bioconjugate could penetrate at least 20 mm of skin tissue, while the fluorescence of the QDs alone could penetrate no more than 10 mm of skin. In addition, little background signal was detected during the luminescence imaging of the QD-Luc8 bioconjugates, whereas strong background autofluorescence was observed during the fluorescence imaging of the CdTe/CdS QDs. These results indicate that self-illuminating QDs can serve as highly sensitive bioprobes for *in vivo* deep tissue imaging and detection.

5. Self-illuminating QDs for Lymph Node Imaging

As mentioned above, self-illuminating QDs can emit red or NIR fluorescence based on BRET without external excitation. This imaging method does not produce autofluorescence and can be used for deep tissue detection. If self-illuminating QDs are introduced for cancer diagnosis imaging, lymph node (LN) mapping, or other *in vivo* targeted imaging, more accurate and abundant information may be obtained compared with that from fluorescence imaging using QDs. To date, self-illuminating nanoparticles have been used for *in vivo* cancer targeted imaging, *in vivo* lymphatic imaging, drug release and cancer therapy [12–15].

In 2011, Kosaka *et al.* [13] used a QD-BRET system for *in vivo* mouse lymphatic imaging. They prepared a QD(655)-Luc8 nanoconjugate that was injected subcutaneously at different sites in mice followed by intravenous coelenterazine injection. The axillary lymphatic duct and LN of a mouse emitted bright fluorescence after QD(655)-Luc8 nanoconjugate was injected into the left paw. This indicated that BRET occurred *in vivo* and QD fluorescence was efficiently excited by the bioluminescence. Imaging of the LNs after resection further demonstrated that a large amount of QD(655)-Luc8 nanoconjugate migrated into the left axillary node and retained bright bioluminescence and fluorescence. When QD(655)-Luc8 nanoconjugate was injected into the chin (5 pmol), an ear (5 pmol) and four paws (10 pmol in each paw), the lymphatic basins and nodes near the injection sites were clearly visualized in the BRET images after intravenous injection of coelenterazine (10 μg). Almost no background signal was detected. Because the concentration of circulating coelenterazine and stability of Luc8 on the QDs decreased over time, the intensity of QD fluorescence based on BRET in the LNs decreased over time and only lasted about 30 min after coelenterazine injections. This is the major disadvantage of BRET imaging using QDs compared with fluorescence imaging using QDs.

Although the luminescence of the self-illuminating QDs in tissue decreased over time, our research group found that the luminescence could be recovered after injection of more luciferase substrate [12], which was illustrated in Fig. 3.9. We subcutaneously injected 80 μL of CdTe/CdS QD-Luc8 (QDs: ~0.5 μmol/L) and 5 μL of coelenterazine (1

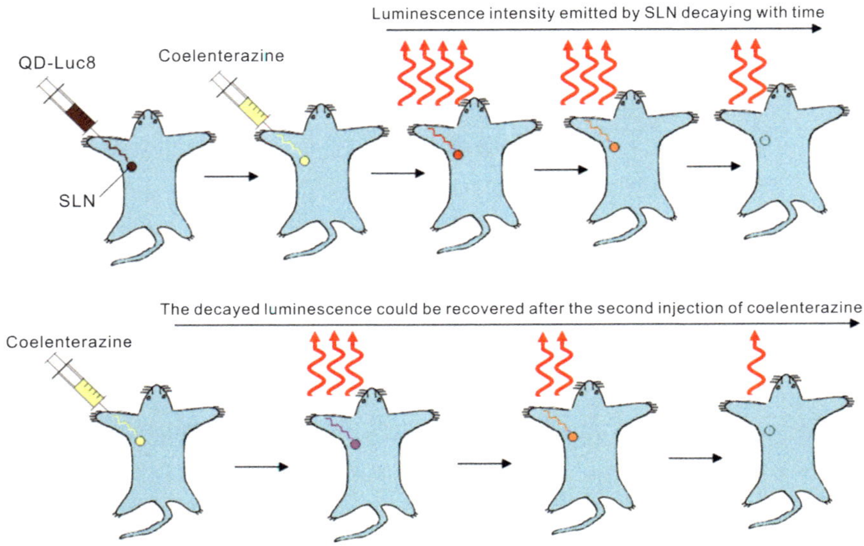

Fig. 3.9. The luminescence generated by the QD-BRET systems trapped within the SLN could be reilluminated by reinjection of the substrate.

μg/μL) into a paw of a nude mouse. Our results showed that the mouse axillary region emitted bright fluorescence (the bioluminescence of Luc8 was filtered) as early as 1 min after injection without external excitation. The *in vivo* axillary LN could be observed easily in real time because only the injection site and axillary region exhibited bright fluorescence; no autobioluminescence was observed elsewhere on the mouse. The fluorescence of QD-Luc8 bioconjugate trapped within the axillary LN persisted for at least 100 min after the injection, which could provide enough time for operators to identify the LN. The persistence time of *in vivo* emission can be tailored by changing the concentrations of QD-Luc8 bioconjugate and coelenterazine. When the BRET signal of QD-Luc8 bioconjugate in the axillary region decayed to close to zero 120 min after injection, the luminescence signal could be recovered when more coelenterazine (5 μL, 1 μg/μL) was intradermally injected into the mouse paw at the same site as the first injection. In addition, the recovered luminescence signal within the LN persisted for at least 50 min. Interestingly, when more coelenterazine was injected into the mouse paw about 5 h after the first injection, the decayed BRET signal from the LN recovered and persisted for about 40 min. We found that the bioactivity of QD-Luc8 bioconjugate in a mouse persisted for no more than 10 h because the BRET signal was difficult to observe after injection of more coelenterazine about 10 h after the first injection. However, when the imaging mode was switched to fluorescence imaging, the strong autofluorescence produced by the liver, stomach, intestines, and skin of the mouse was clearly observed.

6. Discussion

In vivo bioluminescence imaging using red or NIR QD-BRET systems is a novel imaging technique that has attracted considerable attention over the past 10 years. This imaging strategy exhibits great advantages over the fluorescent imaging because the autofluorescence of animal tissue is removed and deep tissue can be imaged. This strategy is also superior to the commonly used bioluminescence imaging and optical imaging based on organic fluorescent dyes (fluorescent proteins or small organic dyes) because the QDs possess excellent optical properties, the difference between the emission peaks of the QDs and luciferase is more than 100 nm, and the efficiency of BRET can exceed 50%. In addition, fluorescent imaging using QDs and bioluminescence imaging using QD-Luc8 can be combined to improve the accuracy of deep tissue detection.

To date, using the self-illuminating semiconductor QDs for *in vivo* cancer target imaging has been seldom reported. This may be because that only weak BRET signal could be detected in tumor site after the tumor-bearing animals were injected with the QD-BRET systems. Although the self-illuminating QDs have been used for drug release and cancer cell killing [15], this technique may be not suitable for *in vivo* long-term cancer therapy.

The bioluminescence of QD-BRET systems in animal tissue is less stable than the fluorescence of QDs. This may be mainly because the amount of luciferase (e.g., Luc8) molecules on the QD surface and substrate (e.g., coelenterazine) molecules in the target tissue decrease over time. Although Luc8 exhibits high stability in animal bodies compared with other luciferases, its bioactivity also decreases over time. These factors are disadvantages for long-term *in vivo* detection. Furthermore, the substrate coelenterazine is expensive, and the expression and purification of Luc8 is complex. In addition, the semiconductor QDs especially the cadmium-containing QDs are toxic to cells and animals [16–23]. Therefore, only when more stable luciferases, inexpensive substrates and low-toxicity QDs are developed in the future is it likely that bioluminescence imaging using QD-BRET systems will be employed in clinical applications.

References

[1] Ghoroghchian PP, Therien MJ and Hammer DA. (2009). *In vivo* fluorescence imaging: a personal perspective. *Wires Nanomed. Nanobi.*, **1**:156–167.

[2] So MK, Xu CJ, Loening AM, Gambhir SS and Rao JH. (2006). Self-illuminating quantum dot conjugates for *in vivo* imaging. *Nat. Biotechnol*, **24**:339–343.

[3] Sadikot RT and Blackwell TS. (2005). Bioluminescence imaging. *Proc. Am. Thorac Soc.*, **2**:537–540, 11–12.

[4] Milligan G. (2004). Applications of bioluminescence- and fluorescence resonance energy transfer to drug discovery at G protein-coupled receptors. *Eur. J. Pharm. Sci.*, **21**:397–405.

[5] Xia ZY and Rao JH. (2009). Biosensing and imaging based on bioluminescence resonance energy transfer. *Curr. Opin. Biotechnol.*, **20**:37–44.

[6] Kumar M, Zhang DH, Broyles D and Deo SK. (2011). A rapid, sensitive, and selective bioluminescence resonance energy transfer (BRET)-based nucleic acid sensing system. *Biosens. Bioelectro.*, **30**:133–139.

[7] Banaszynski LA, Liu CW and Wandless TJ. (2005). Characterization of the FKBP. rapamycin. FRB ternary complex. *J. Am. Chem. Soc.*, **127**: 4715–4721.

[8] Dragulescu-Andrasi A, Chan CT, De A, Massoud TF and Gambhir SS. (2011). Bioluminescence resonance energy transfer (BRET) imaging of protein-protein interactions within deep tissues of living subjects. *PNAS.* **108**:12060–12065.

[9] Yao HQ, Zhang Y, Xiao F, Xia ZY and Rao JH. (2007). Quantum dot/bioluminescence resonance energy transfer based highly sensitive detection of proteases. *Angew. Chem. Int. Edit.*, **46**:4346–4349.

[10] Xia ZY, Xing Y, So MK, Koh AL, Sinclair R and Rao JH. (2008). Multiplex Detection of Protease Activity with Quantum Dot Nanosensors Prepared by Intein-Mediated Specific Bioconjugation. *Anal. Chem.*, **80**:8649–8655.

[11] Xing Y, So MK, Koh AL, Sinclair R and Rao JH. (2008). Improved QD-BRET conjugates for detection and imaging. *Biochem. Biophys. Res. Commun.*, **372**:388–394.

[12] Wu Q and Chu MQ. (2012). Self-illuminating quantum dots for highly sensitive *in vivo* real-time luminescent mapping of sentinel lymph nodes. *Int J Nanomed.*, **7**:3433–3443.

[13] Kosaka N, Mitsunaga M, Bhattacharyya S, Miller SC, Choyke PL and Kobayashi H. (2011). Self-illuminating *in vivo* lymphatic imaging using a bioluminescence resonance energy transfer quantum dot nano-particle. *Contrast Media Mol I.*, **6**:55–59.

[14] Xiong LQ, Shuhendler AJ and Rao JH. (2012). Self-luminescing BRET-FRET near-infrared dots for *in vivo* lymph-node mapping and tumour imaging. *Nat. Commun.*, **3**:1193.

[15] Song WC, Shin SW, Park KS, Jang MS, Choi JH, Oh BK and Um SH. (2015). Self-illuminative cascade-reaction-driven anticancer therapeutic cassettes made of cooperatively interactive nanocomplexes. *Colloids Surf B.*, **126**:580–584.

[16] Su YY, Peng F, Jiang ZY, Zhong YL, Lu YM, Jiang XX, Huang Q, Fan C, Lee ST and He Y. (2011). *In vivo* distribution, pharmacokinetics, and toxicity of aqueous synthesized cadmium-containing quantum dots. *Biomaterials*, **32**:5855–5862.

[17] Kusic H and Leszczynska D. (2012). Altered toxicity of organic pollutants in water originated from simultaneous exposure to UV photolysis and CdSe/ZnS quantum dots. *Chemosphere*, **89**:900–906.

[18] Ambrosone A, Mattera L, Marchesano V, Quarta A, Susha AS, Tino A, Rogach AL and Tortiglione C. (2012). Mechanisms underlying toxicity induced by CdTe quantum dots determined in an invertebrate model organism. *Biomaterials*, **33**:1991–2000.

[19] Fang TT, Li X, Wang QS, Zhang ZJ, Liu P and Zhang CC. (2012). Toxicity evaluation of CdTe quantum dots with different size on *Escherichia coli*. *Toxicol In Vitro*, **26**:1233–1239.

[20] Peng L, He M, Chen BB, Wu QM, Zhang ZL, Pang DW, Zhu Y and Hu B. (2013). Cellular uptake, elimination and toxicity of CdSe/ZnS quantum dots in HepG2 cells. *Biomaterials*, **34**:9545–9558.

[21] Tang Y, Han SL, Liu HM, Chen X, Huang L, Li XH and Zhang T. (2013). The role of surface chemistry in determining *in vivo* biodistribution and toxicity of CdSe/ZnS core-shell quantum dots. *Biomaterials*, **34**: 8741–8755.

[22] Liu T, Xing R, Zhou YF, Zhang J, Su YY, Zhang KQ He Y, Sima YH and Xu SQ. (2014). Hematopoiesis toxicity induced by CdTe quantum dots determined in an invertebrate model organism. *Biomaterials*, **35**: 2942–2951.

[23] Kauffer FA, Merlin C, Balan L and Schneider R. (2014). Incidence of the core composition on the stability, the ROS production and the toxicity of CdSe quantum dots. *J. Hazard Mater.*, **268**:246–255.

Chapter 4

Semiconductor Quantum Rods with Bright Fluorescence and Slow Bleaching Kinetics for Cell Labeling and *In Vivo* Imaging

Semiconductor nanocrystals include zero-dimensional spherical quantum dots (QDs) and one-dimensional semiconductor quantum rods (QRs) and quantum wires (QWs). Both QDs and QRs have received extensive attention in biomedical research because of their interesting optical properties, including bright and stable size-dependent fluorescence and other unique optical properties such as narrow symmetric fluorescent emission spectra. However, the optical properties of QRs make them better fluorescent probes for *in vitro* and *in vivo* biomedical imaging than QDs. For example, QRs have brighter fluorescence with slower photobleaching than QDs. Therefore, QRs are suitable for long-term fluorescence imaging. In addition, QRs have a larger surface area than QDs for conjugating biomolecules, which allows QR bioconjugates to exhibit stronger functions than QD ones. In this chapter, the optical properties, cell labeling and imaging applications, and ability to penetrate physiological barriers of QRs are described. The use of QR-bioluminescence resonance energy transfer (BRET) systems using QRs as energy acceptors and the toxicity of QRs are also discussed.

1. Introduction

In general, spherical nanoparticles form more readily than other shapes like rods. Spherical semiconductor QDs are the most common inorganic fluorescent dyes. Most researchers may only synthesize and use spherical QDs in their studies. However, the nonspherical nanoparticles usually exhibit peculiar properties compared with the spherical nanoparticles.

Recently, besides the zero-dimensional semiconductor QDs described in the previous chapters, one-dimensional semiconductor QRs and QWs also have been paid considerable attention. Both QRs and QWs have unique optical properties, but the size of QRs is ranging from 2 to 10 nm in width and from 5 to 100 nm in length, which is obviously shorter than the QWs. Therefore, QRs have been attracting significant interest in biomedical research areas. QRs composed of cadmium selenide (CdSe), lead selenide, indium phosphide and indium arsenide, as well as core–shell QRs with structures such as CdSe/cadmium sulfide (CdS), CdSe/CdS/zinc sulfide (ZnS), and cadmium telluride selenide ($CdTe_xSe_{1-x}$/ZnS have been reported in recent years. These rod-shaped nanoparticles can be synthesized by solution techniques using organometallic precursors [1, 2], micellar templating techniques [3], microwave techniques [4], a solution–liquid–solid method [5, 6], a seeded-growth method [7] ,and biosynthesis (e.g., using *Aspergillus terreus*) [8].

Semiconductor QRs have brighter fluorescence, larger absorption cross sections and slower bleaching kinetics than QDs. This helps to reduce the toxicity of QRs to cells and animals because a low dosage of QRs may emit very bright fluorescence for a long time. To date, QRs have been used for *in vitro* cell labeling and *in vivo* tumor-targeted imaging.

2. Optical Properties of Semiconductor QRs

QRs have similar optical properties to QDs in terms of broad absorption, and narrow symmetric emission that is bright and stable. It was mentioned in Chapter 1 that zero-dimensional QDs show size-tunable broad absorption. The optical properties of one-dimensional QRs are also size dependent.

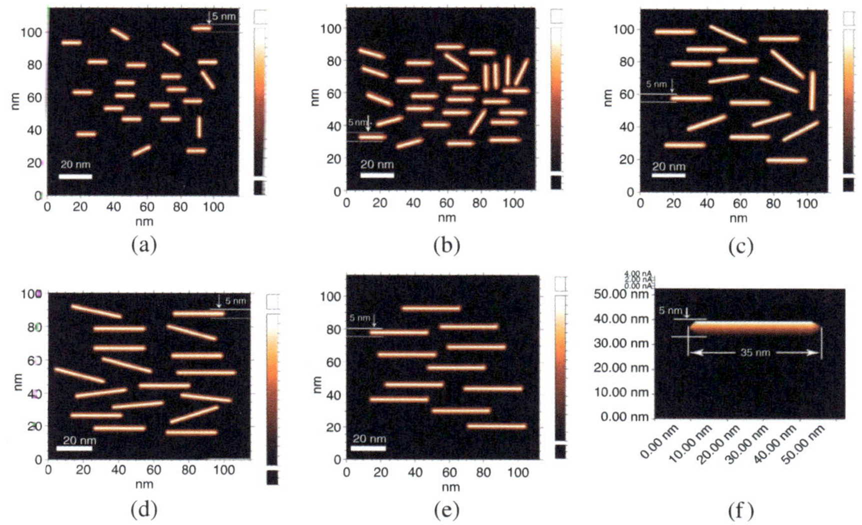

Fig. 4.1. STM images of CdSe QRs with a fixed width of 5 nm and lengths of (a) 12.5 nm, (b) 17.5 nm, (c) 25 nm, (d) 30 nm, and (e) 35 nm. (f) Three-dimensional image. Reprinted with permission from Ref. [9]. Copyright (2009) Elsevier.

As strongly quantum-confined nanostructures, the energy band-gap between the valence and conduction bands of QRs, which can be determined easily from their ultraviolet-visible (UV-vis) absorption spectrum, changes with rod size. Talaat *et al.* [9] investigated the energy band gaps of a series of CdSe QRs of different sizes (different length and diameter) using scanning tunneling microscopy (STM) and optical spectroscopy techniques at room temperature. They selected 10 samples with different morphologies to study the relationship between the absorption spectra and size of the CdSe QRs. The first set contained five samples with a fixed width of 5 nm and lengths of 12.5, 17.5, 25, 30 and 35 nm (Fig. 4.1). The second set consisted of five samples with a fixed length of 20 nm and widths of 3.5, 4, 4.25, 4.5 and 5 nm (Fig. 4.2). The first set of samples all exhibited a sharp absorption peak at about 555 nm with no obvious shift as the QR length increased from 12.5 to 35 nm (Fig. 4.3a). This suggests that the optical absorption of QRs does not depend on QR length. This is because the energy gap of the first set of samples (2.23 ± 0.01 eV) with different lengths is constant.

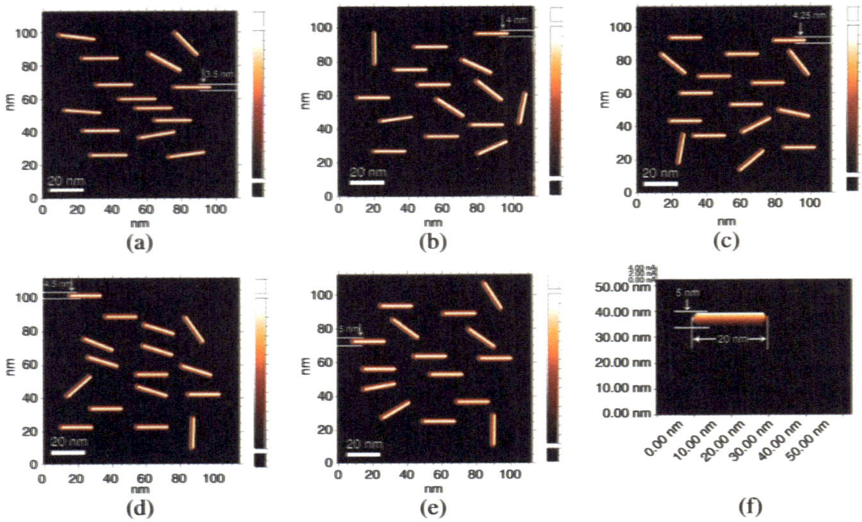

Fig. 4.2. STM images of CdSe QRs with a fixed length of 20 nm and widths of (a) 3.5 nm, (b) 4 nm, (c) 4.25 nm, (d) 4.5 nm and (e) 5 nm (f) Three-dimensional image. Reprinted with permission from Ref. [9]. Copyright (2009) Elsevier.

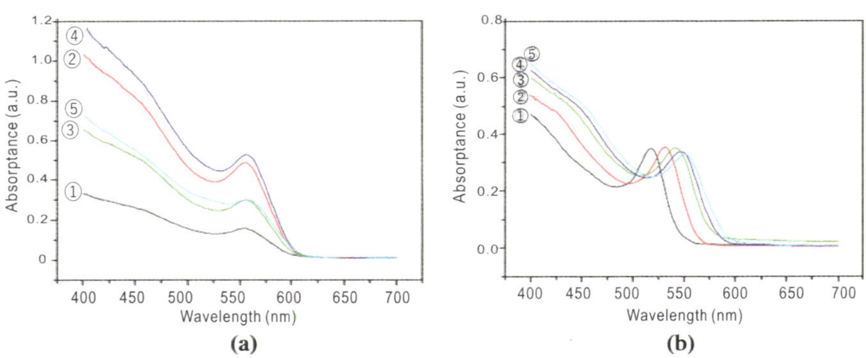

Fig. 4.3. Optical absorption spectra of CdSe QRs. (a) QRs with a fixed width of 5 nm and different lengths. ① 12.5 nm, ② 17.5 nm, ③ 25 nm, ④ 30 nm, and ⑤ 35 nm. (b) QRs with a fixed length of 20 nm and different widths. ① 3.5 nm, ② 4 nm, ③ 4.25 nm, ④ 4.5 nm and ⑤ 5 nm. Reprinted with permission from Ref. [9]. Copyright (2009) Elsevier.

Conversely, the absorption peaks of the second set of samples exhibit an obvious red shift as the QR width is increased from 3.5 to 5 nm (Fig. 4.3b). The red shift of the absorption peak is caused by the energy gap decreasing from 2.39 ± 0.01 to 2.22 ± 0.01 eV as the QR width increases from 3.5 to 5 nm.

Compared with QDs, QRs have a bigger Stokes shift, which is the difference between absorption and emission maxima. Figure 4.4a shows the morphology of CdTe QRs at different stages during their formation [10]. The low-aspect-ratio QRs evolved into nanorods with higher aspect ratios and then to spheres. The Stokes shifts of these samples increases as the rods lengthen, then decreases as ripening occurs (Fig. 4.4b), which indicates that the Stokes shift is controlled by the aspect ratio of the QRs [10]. This observation also reveals that the fluorescence of QRs red shifts with increasing rod size.

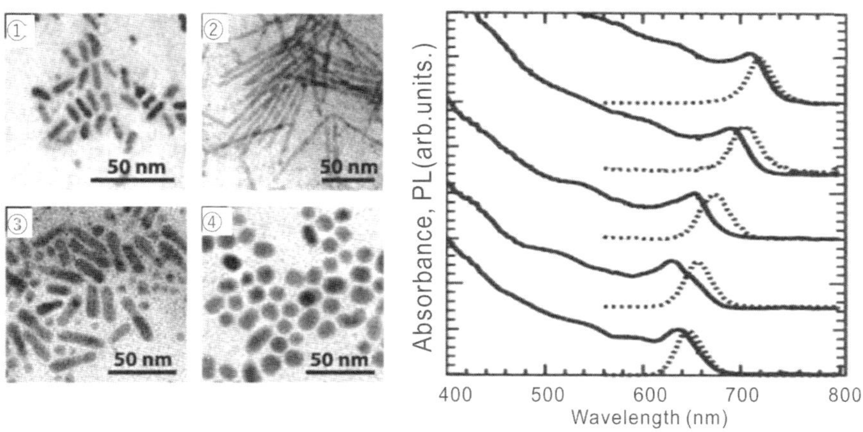

(a) (b)

Fig. 4.4. (a) Evolution of the size and shape of CdTe nanorods. After two sequential injections, nanorods with a low aspect ratio form, as in ①. Further sequential injections elongate the nanorods to achieve aspect ratios greater than 10 ②. Upon further heating, the rods undergo a shape transition to form spheres, initially increasing in diameter while decreasing in length ③ and ultimately reshaping into spheres ④. (b) Absorbance (solid lines) and photoluminescence (PL) (dotted lines) of CdTe nanocrystal aliquots taken during QR growth (excitation wavelength = 560 nm). Reprinted with permission from Ref. [10]. Copyright (2005) American Chemical Society.

In addition, the fluorescence from a single QR is brighter than that from a QD and has slower bleaching kinetics [11, 12]. QRs also have a larger absorption cross section [13], and faster radiative decay rate than those of QDs [14]. A single QR exhibits linearly polarized emission unlike the plane-polarized light from a single QD [15]. The emission of a single QR can be reversibly switched on and off by an external electric field [11, 16].

3. QRs for Cell Labeling and Imaging

As mentioned above, QRs have unique optical properties that differ from those of QDs. Researchers are paying increasing attention to the use of QRs in biomedical applications. In early 2007, Fu *et al.* [11] used QRs in cell imaging research. They coated CdSe/CdS/ZnS core/shell QRs (CdS/ZnS graded shell on CdSe QRs) with silane molecules (Fig. 4.5a) to transfer the QRs from organic solvent into aqueous solution and render them biofunctional. They found that the silanized QRs remained well dispersed in aqueous buffer for over two years. To compare QRs and QDs in cell imaging, they selected silanized CdSe/CdS/ZnS QRs and QDs (Figs. 4.5b and 4.5c, respectively) with the same fluorescence wavelength (emission maxima: 593 nm) and quantum yield (9%) (Fig. 4.5d) for specific cancer cell labeling and studying fluorescence signals in cells at the single-molecule level. The silanized QRs did not obviously disturb the physiological functions of cells, including cell division and migration. After being conjugated with a peptide (Chariot), the resulting QR bioconjugate could penetrate through the membrane of cancer cells (MDA-MB-231) and accumulate near the nucleus (Fig. 4.5e). Even after the cancer cells were incubated with the QR bioconjugate for 24 h, the cells still looked healthy (Fig. 4.5e).

Fu and colleagues found that the QRs allowed single-molecule fluorescence imaging with higher sensitivity than the QDs [11]. Because analysis of single-molecule kinetic and dynamic behavior in living cells is challenging, using the unique optical properties of QRs to improve the level of tracking of single molecules in living cells may be very important. Figures 4.6a and 4.6b reveal that the fluorescence signal of the QRs is markedly stronger than that of the QDs under the same excitation and

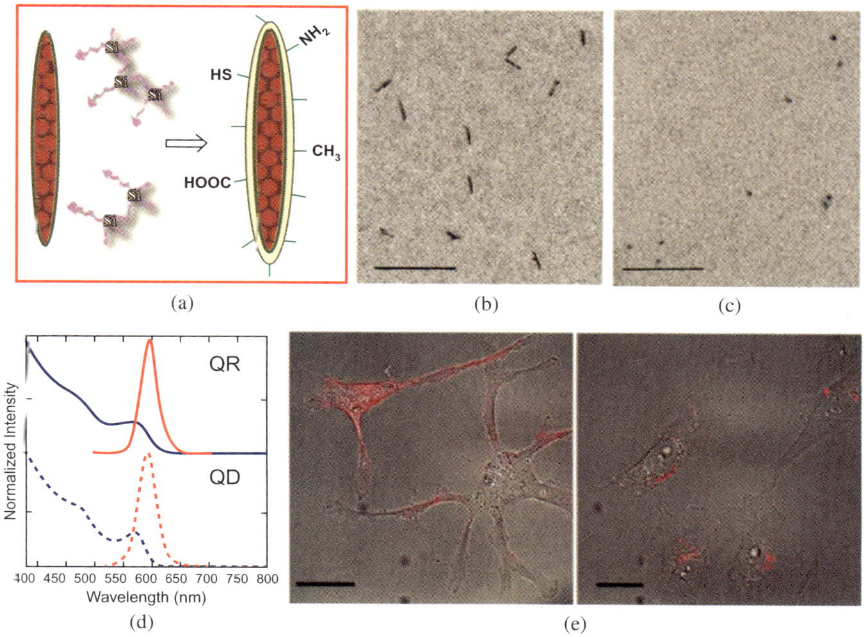

Fig. 4.5. Silanized CdSe/CdS/ZnS QRs for cell imaging. (a) Schematic illustration of silanization of QRs. Transmission electron microscopy (TEM) images of (b) silanized QRs and (c) QDs in neutral phosphate buffer (scale bar: 100 nm). (d) UV-vis absorption and emission spectra of silanized QRs and QDs. (e) Human breast cancer cells MDA-MB-231 incubated with the silanized QR- Chariot bioconjugate for 1 h (left) and 24 h (right) (scale bar: 20 μm). Reprinted with permission from Ref. [11]. Copyright (2007) American Chemical Society.

detection conditions. The signal-to-noise ratio of QR fluorescence is obviously higher than that of QD fluorescence (Fig. 4.6c). Fu and co-workers then introduced a small amount of silanized QRs and QDs into MDA-MB-231 cancer cells using streptolysin-O, a protein that generates holes in cell membranes. They found that the QR fluorescence remained bright inside living cells, whereas single QDs were not observed inside the cells (Fig. 4.6d). This indicates that single QR fluorescence is brighter and more stable than that from a single QD. Overall, QRs show great potential for long-term detection and tracking single molecules within living cells.

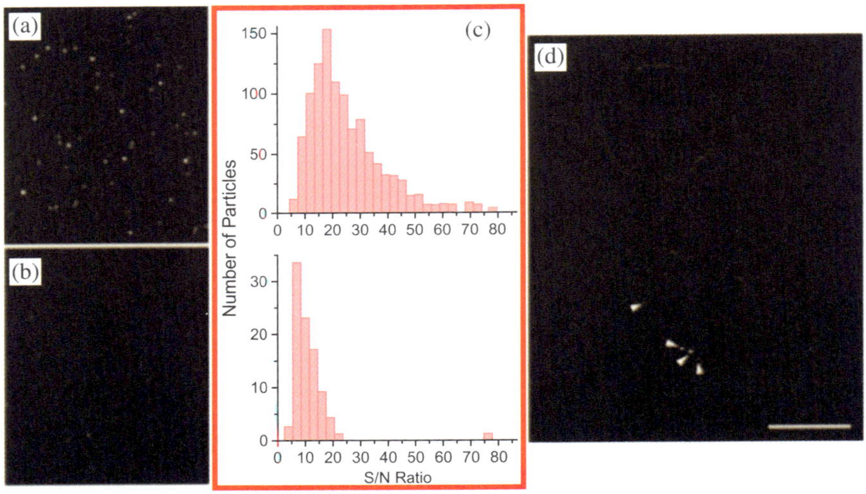

Fig. 4.6. Comparison of fluorescent imaging using QRs and QDs at the single-molecule level. Fluorescent signal of (a) QRs and (b) QDs. (c) Signal-to-noise (S/N) ratio of QRs (top) and QDs (bottom). (d) Single QRs (indicated by arrows) inside live MDA-MB-231 cells. The scale bar is 10 μm. Reprinted with permission from Ref. [11]. Copyright (2007) American Chemical Society.

Also in 2007, Yong *et al.* [17] reported live cell imaging using antibody-conjugated CdSe/CdS/ZnS QRs (CdS/ZnS graded shell on CdSe QRs) as targeted optical probes. The QRs were coated with mercaptoundecanoic acid and lysine when they were transferred from organic to aqueous solution. The morphologies of the QRs are shown in Fig. 4.7. Because transferrin receptor (TfR) is overexpressed in cancer cells, to specifically target binding cancer cells, Yong and co-workers conjugated transferrin (Tf) onto the surfaces of the QRs to form a QR-Tf bioconjugate. Figure 4.8 shows HeLa cells (cervical cancer cells that overexpress TfR) after incubation with the QR-Tf bioconjugate and controls. Only the cancer cells treated with QR-Tf emit bright fluorescence. Conversely, for the two control experiments where HeLa cells were incubated with QRs without Tf or saturated with free Tf for 2 h before treatment with QR-Tf, only a small amount of QRs was observed on the cell surfaces. These results further demonstrate that QR-based bioconjugates can be used as fluorescent bioprobes for targeted labeling and imaging.

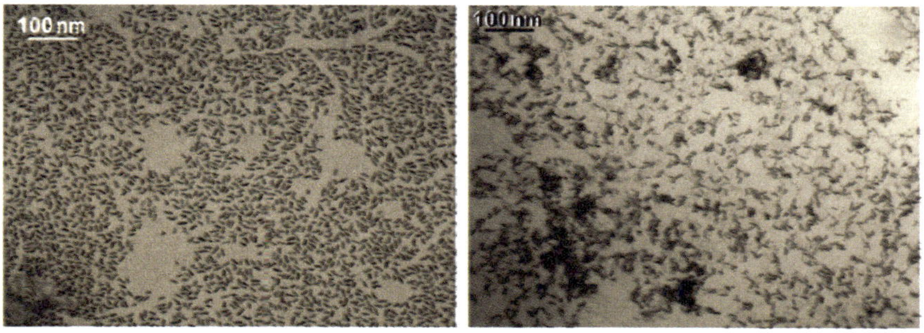

(a) (b)

Fig. 4.7. TEM images of CdSe/CdS/ZnS QRs deposited from (a) organic media and (b) aqueous media. Reprinted with permission from Ref. [17]. Copyright (2007) American Chemical Society.

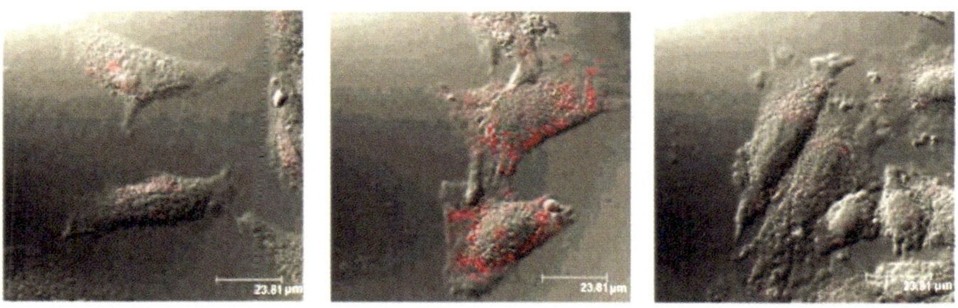

(a) (b) (c)

Fig. 4.8. HeLa cells incubated with (a) lysine-coated CdSe/CdS/ZnS QRs. (b, c) Tf-conjugated CdSe/CdS/ZnS QRs. Cells in (c) were saturated with free Tf for 2 h to block the available TfR on the cell surface before treatment with QR-Tf. The red areas in each panel are QR fluorescence. Reprinted with permission from Ref. [17]. Copyright (2007) American Chemical Society.

Simultaneously identifying the overexpressed receptors on cancer cell surfaces is an important technique for rapid diagnosis of tumors. Because semiconductor QRs have bright and stable fluorescence, these nanomaterials may have great potential for this application. In 2008, Yong *et al.* [18] synthesized two types of CdSe/CdS/ZnS QRs (CdS/ZnS graded shell on CdSe QRs) for the multiplex labeling of live human cancer cells. The first was orange-emitting CdSe/CdS/ZnS QRs (band-edge emission: 610 nm) with dimensions of 4 × 14 nm, and the second was red-emitting

CdSe/CdS/ZnS QRs (band-edge emission: 657 nm) with dimensions of 6.5 × 26 nm. The QRs were conjugated with Tf, then used to label human nasopharyngeal epidermal carcinoma (KB) cells. Bright fluorescence from both types of QRs were simultaneously observed in cells. They also conjugated folic acid (FA) onto the red-emitting QRs. The KB cells were then incubated with both these red-emitting FA-conjugated QRs and orange-emitting ones conjugated with Tf. They found that the cancer cells were co-labeled with the two different colored QRs, which could be observed clearly by fluorescence imaging. Control experiments demonstrated that the KB cells were labeled with the QR bioconjugates through specific receptor-mediated uptake. The same group also conjugated various biomolecules including anti-Claudin 4, anti-mesothelin and mouse-anti-IgG onto the orange- and red-emitting QRs for multiplex labeling of human pancreatic cancer cells (Panc-1). This work suggests that multicolored QR bioconjugates may be useful as efficient optical tracking probes for rapid cancer diagnosis.

To improve the quantum yield of QRs and reduce their toxicity, Deka *et al.* [12] synthesized CdSe/CdS/ZnS QRs with a double shell. They fabricated "dot-in-a-rod" CdSe QD/CdS QR core/shell nanocrystals, then coated the CdSe/CdS QRs with a ZnS shell (Fig. 4.9a). The structure of

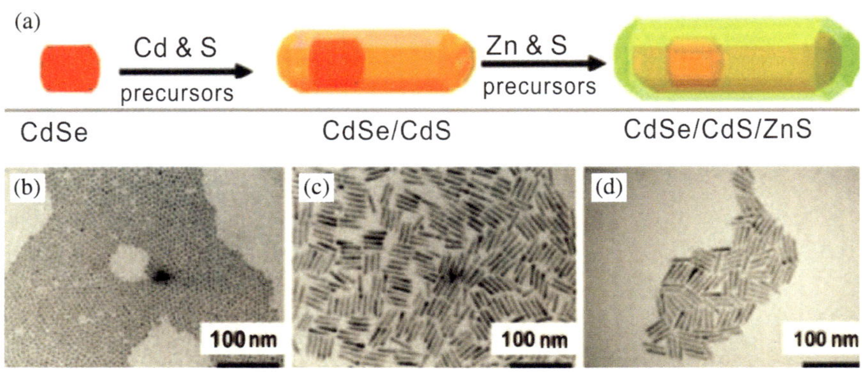

Fig. 4.9. (a) Schematic illustration of the formation of double-shell CdSe/CdS/ZnS QRs. TEM images of (b) starting CdSe cores, (c) CdSe/CdS QRs, and (d) CdSe/CdS/ZnS QRs. Reprinted with permission from Ref. [12]. Copyright (2009) American Chemical Society.

such double-shell CdSe/CdS/ZnS QRs is different from that of QRs with a CdSe QR core and CdS/ZnS graded shell. In these double-shell QRs, the CdSe core was spherical with a diameter of ~3.5 nm, the starting CdSe/CdS QRs were 5 × 24 nm, and the final CdSe/CdS/ZnS QRs were 6 × 26 nm (Fig. 4.9b–d). The quantum yield of these novel CdSe/CdS/ZnS QRs could reach up to 75%, whereas those of the starting CdSe/CdS QRs and CdSe QD cores were only about 50% and 15%, respectively. In addition, the toxicity of the CdSe/CdS/ZnS QRs was obviously reduced compared with that of the CdSe/CdS QRs or CdSe QDs; covering the CdSe/CdS QRs with a ZnS shell decreased their cell toxicity by 20%. This is because the ZnS shell inhibited the release of cadmium (Cd) from the QR surface. To compare the cell imaging abilities of the QRs and QDs, polymer (the outer layer was amine-terminated polyethylene glycol (PEG))-coated CdSe/CdS/ZnS QRs, CdSe/CdS QRs and CdSe/CdS QDs were incubated with HeLa cells for 24 h with the same Cd concentration of 50 μM. Following this treatment, all cells emitted bright fluorescence (Figs. 4.10a–4.10f), and the cells labeled with CdSe/CdS/ZnS QRs were the brightest. This is because the fluorescence of the CdSe/CdS/ZnS QRs is brighter than that of the other two types of nanoparticles. Fluorescence spectra of different cell suspensions showed that the fluorescence intensity of the cells incubated with CdSe/CdS/ZnS QRs was about three times higher than that of the cells incubated with CdSe/CdS QDs (Fig. 4.10g). This further indicates that the fluorescence of a single QR is brighter than that of a QD, and that it is not easily quenched in cells, which is beneficial for long-term biomedical imaging.

4. Ability of QRs to Penetrate Physiological Barriers

For nanoparticles to accumulate at a target site *in vivo*, they need to penetrate through many physiological barriers including a large amount of intercellular spaces from the injection site to the target tissue. Therefore, nanocarriers should migrate readily through tissues for efficient targeted diagnostic imaging and therapy. The blood–brain barrier (BBB) is a dynamic barrier that protects the brain against invading organisms and unwanted substances [19]. Although numerous candidate drugs can effectively treat brain or central nervous system diseases *in vitro*, these

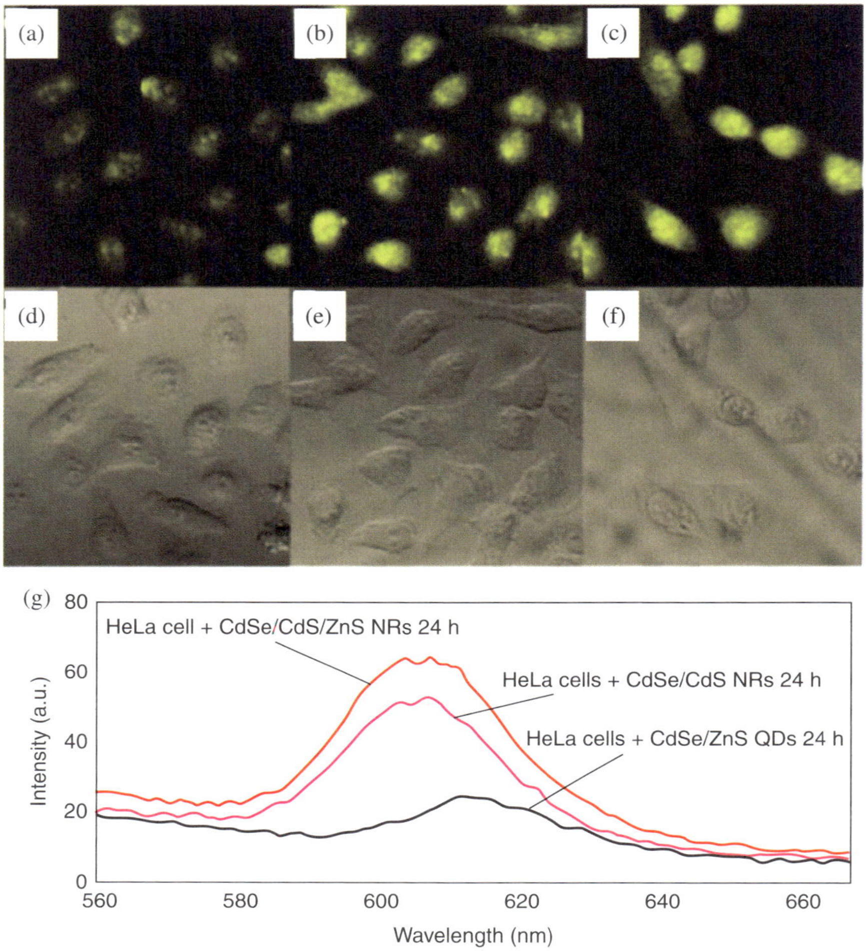

Fig. 4.10. HeLa cells incubated with (a, d) CdSe/ZnS QDs, (b, e) CdSe/CdS core–shell QRs, and (c, f) double-shell CdSe/CdS/ZnS QRs for 24 h with the same Cd concentration. (g) Fluorescence spectra of different cell suspensions (each containing the same number of cells). PL intensities were normalized to the number of cells. Reprinted with permission from Ref. [12]. Copyright (2009) American Chemical Society.

drugs usually exhibit low efficacy *in vivo* because many drugs cannot penetrate the BBB. To improve the efficiency of targeted delivery of drugs across the BBB, researchers have developed numerous novel nanocarriers, peptides and antibodies to aid drug transport. In addition, novel imaging

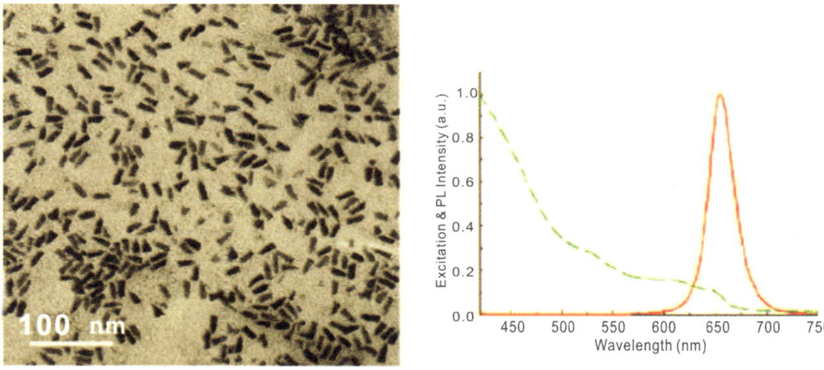

(a) (b)

Fig. 4.11. (a) TEM image and (b) absorption and emission spectra of red-emitting CdSe/CdS/ZnS QRs. Reprinted with permission from Ref. [20]. Copyright (2008) American Chemical Society.

methods to efficiently monitor drug molecules penetrating across the BBB are also useful. The small size and stable fluorescence of QRs mean they have potential for tracking drug delivery *in vivo*.

In 2008, Xu *et al.* [20] used QR bioconjugates as efficient targeted fluorescent probes for transmigration across the BBB. They conjugated Tf antibodies onto red-emitting CdSe/CdS/ZnS QRs with dimensions of 6.5 × 26 nm (Fig. 4.11). The resulting QR-Tf bioconjugate was used to investigate how biomolecules were delivered across an *in vitro* BBB model. The *in vitro* BBB model consisted of two-compartment wells in a culture plate. They added different concentrations the QR-Tf bioconjugate into the upper chamber of wells in the model and incubated the model for different periods. When the QD-Tf bioconjugate was incubated in the BBB model for 6, 26, and 42 h, the uptake of Tf-QR by both upper and lower cell layers increased with the incubation time, which was observed clearly by QR fluorescence. This indicated that the QR-Tf bioconjugate could penetrate through the BBB model through a kinetic process. A control experiment where unconjugated QRs were incubated in the model demonstrated that the migration of the QR-Tf bioconjugate was driven by a receptor-mediated process. The amount of QR-Tf that crossed the *in vitro* BBB also depended on QR-Tf concentration. Figure 4.12 reveals that when ~0.56, 2.3, and 9.2 pmol of QR-Tf bioconjugate were incubated in the BBB model for 26 h, the red fluorescence from both the upper and

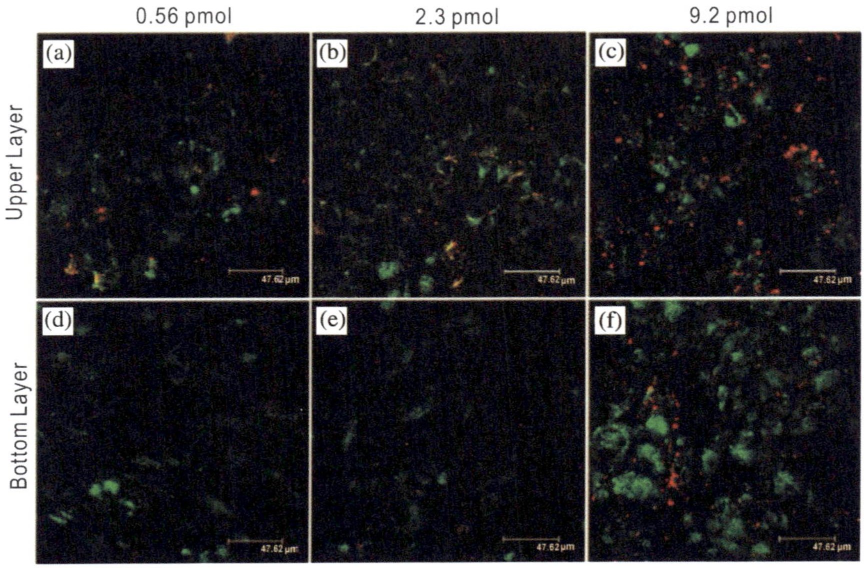

Fig. 4.12. Fluorescence images of the upper and bottom layers of a BBB model incubated with ~0.56, 2.3 and 9.2 pmol of QR-Tf bioconjugate. The red fluorescence represents emission from QR-Tf (QR maximum emission: 658 nm). Reprinted with permission from Ref. [20]. Copyright (2008) American Chemical Society.

lower cell layers increased with bioconjugate concentration. These results confirm that more QR-Tf migrated across the barrier when the QR-Tf concentration was higher.

The passive diffusion of nanoparticles through tissue cells may be markedly less efficient than their active transport. For example, Tf receptor (TfR) is highly localized on the endothelial surfaces of the brain, while Claudin 4 antigen exhibits lower targeting efficiency in the brain than TfR. Xu *et al*. [20] conjugated the anti-Claudin 4 antibody onto orange-emitting QR, then used the resulting orange-emitting QR-bioconjugate and a red-emitting QD-Tf bioconjugate to investigate the difference in targeting specificity between the anti-Claudin 4 antibody and Tf on cells, as well as the abilities of the antibody and Tf to penetrate across the physiological barrier. After both bioconjugates were incubated in the BBB model for 26 h, they found that the uptake of QR-Tf bioconjugate was three times higher than that of the QR- antibody one in the lower layer of the model.

5. QRs for *In Vivo* Fluorescence Imaging

In vivo solid tumor fluorescence imaging is an interesting technique that has great potential for cancer diagnosis. As mentioned above, Tf-conjugated QRs can efficiently penetrate through the BBB via receptor-mediated uptake. It has also been demonstrated above that the optical properties of QRs have advantages over those of QDs. These factors imply that QR bioconjugates may be useful for *in vivo* tumor-targeted imaging.

In 2009, Yong *et al.* [21] demonstrated that CdSe/CdS/ZnS QRs conjugated with cyclic RGD (cRGD) peptide could be successfully used for *in vivo* tumor targeting and imaging in mice. These functionalized QRs were not only conjugated with RGD peptide, but also coated with PEGylated phospholipid micelles (Fig. 4.13). This nonimmunogenic PEG layer improved the dispersion of the QRs in aqueous solution, and also prevented the capture of nanoparticles by the reticuloendothelial system *in vivo*. The obtained QR/PEG/cRGD bioconjugate emitted strong red fluorescence. The researchers injected 1 mg of QR/PEG/cRGD bioconjugate into the tail veins of Panc-1 tumor-bearing mice. These tumors were relatively large, with a volume of about 0.5–0.9 cm^3. The accumulation of the bioconjugate in the tumors could be clearly observed in real time

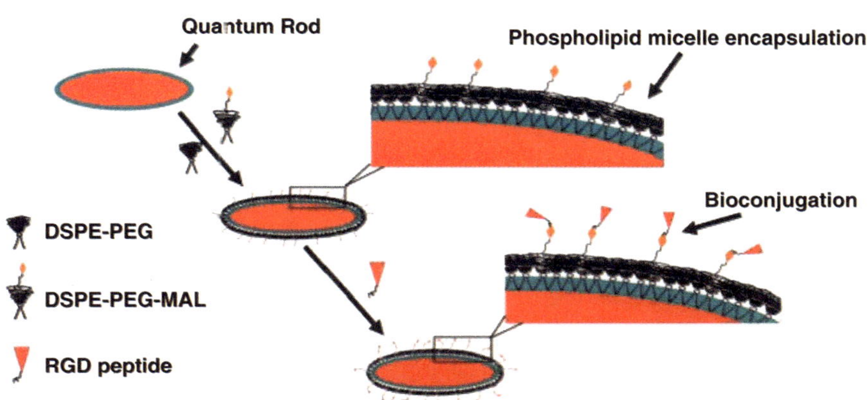

Fig. 4.13. Schematic Illustration of the formation of a QR/PEG/cRGD bioconjugate. Reprinted with permission from Ref. [21]. Copyright (2009) American Chemical Society.

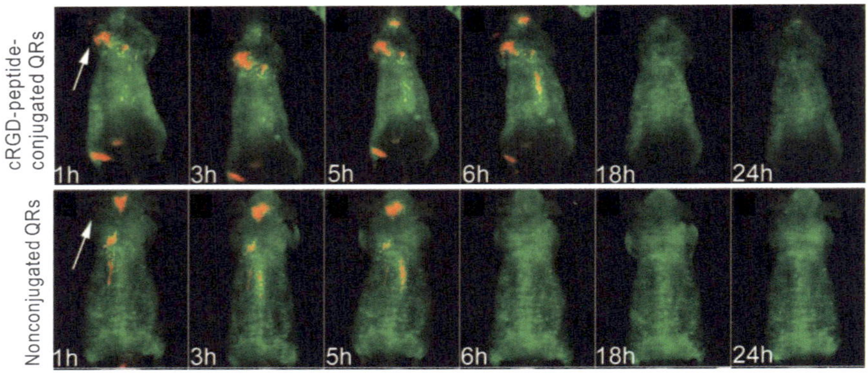

Fig. 4.14. *In vivo* tumor-targeted imaging using a QR/PEG/cRGD bioconjugate (upper images) and QR/PEG control (lower images). The animal model was nude mice bearing large Panc-1 tumors (left shoulder, indicated by white arrows) with a volume of about 0.5–0.9 cm^3. Reprinted with permission from Ref. [21]. Copyright (2009) American Chemical Society.

through the QR fluorescence without resecting the mouse skin and muscle. *In vivo* imaging showed that the tumors emitted bright fluorescence during the initial 6 h post-injection, while nearly no QR fluorescence could be detected 18 h after injection (Fig. 4.14, upper panels). In contrast, QR fluorescence was difficult to discern in the tumors of mice that were intravenously injected with QR/PEG without the cRGD peptide (Fig. 4.14, lower panels).

Yong and colleagues [21] also investigated whether the QR/PEG/cRGD bioconjugate could be used for small tumor target imaging. A nude mouse was inoculated in its right shoulder with $(2–3) \times 10^6$ Panc-1 cells, incubated for 2 weeks, and then injected in its tail vein with ~0.5 mg of QR/PEG/cRGD bioconjugate. Images of the mouse are depicted in Fig. 4.15. The tumor size was significant smaller than that shown in Fig. 4.14. The tumor exhibited strong QR fluorescence after injection, similar to that observed for larger tumors. These results suggest that QR bioconjugates may be used as sensitive fluorescent probes for early cancer diagnosis.

Because the CdSe/CdS/ZnS QRs described above contain Cd, their toxicity should be seriously considered. The Cd toxicity may be reduced by coating the QRs with a hard shell before biomedical use.

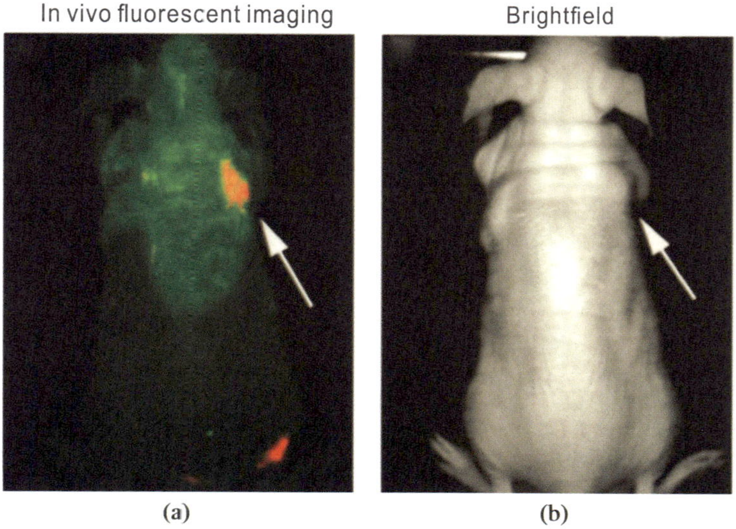

Fig. 4.15. *In vivo* tumor-targeted imaging using a QR/PEG/cRGD bioconjugate. The animal model was a nude mouse bearing a small Panc-1 tumor (right shoulder, indicated by white arrows). The tumor volume was no more than ~0.5 cm^3. Reprinted with permission from Ref. [21]. Copyright (2009) American Chemical Society.

In 2010, Kumar *et al.* [22] encapsulated CdSe/CdS/ZnS QRs with a silica shell (Fig. 4.16). The resulting QR/SiO_2 core–shell nanocomposites emitted bright red fluorescence (maximum emission: 650 nm) with a quantum yield close to 7%. The silica shell could also maintain the fluorescence and colloidal stability of the QRs in aqueous solution. After the QR/SiO_2 nanocomposite (2.5 μg/mL) was incubated with Panc-1 cells (pancreatic cancer cells) and RAW264.7 cells (mouse leukemic monocyte macrophage cells) for 24 h, a large amount of the nanorods migrated into both types of cells via endocytosis without conjugation of specific targeting biomolecules (Fig. 4.17). All cells emitted bright fluorescence without morphological damage even after 24 h of incubation, which indicated that the QR/SiO_2 nanocomposite possessed low toxicity and was suitable for long-term biomedical imaging. Kumar and co-workers then intratumorally injected the QR/SiO_2 nanocomposite (50 μL, 2 mg/mL) into mice bearing Panc-1 tumors. Bright fluorescence emitted by the QR/SiO_2 nanocomposite was observed from the tumor tissues through the skin, and the

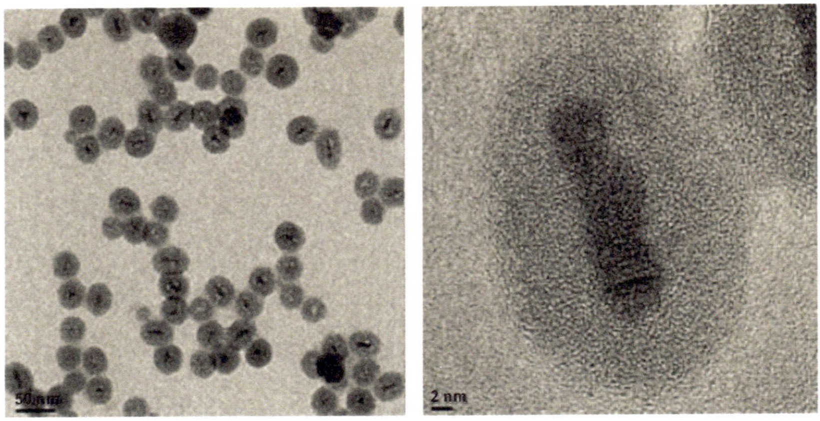

(a) (b)

Fig. 4.16. (a) Low- and (b) high-resolution TEM images of silica-coated CdSe/CdS/ZnS QRs. Reprinted with permission from Ref. [22]. Copyright (2010) American Chemical Society.

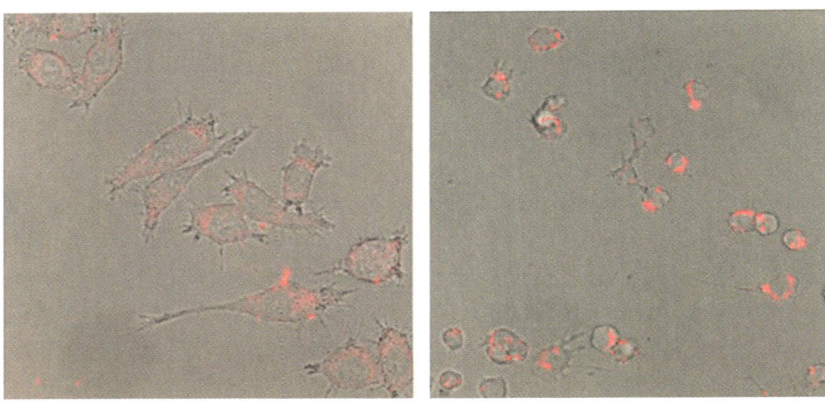

(a) (b)

Fig. 4.17. Fluorescence images of (a) Panc-1 and (b) RAW264.7 cells incubated with QR/SiO_2 (2.5 μg/mL) for 24 h. Reprinted with permission from Ref. [22]. Copyright (2010) American Chemical Society.

nanorods moved to the tumor region and remained localized there, which was detected in real time by *in vivo* imaging (Fig. 4.18). This indicates that the QR/SiO_2 bioconjugate can retain stable fluorescence in the tumor tissue of living animals, making it suitable for *in vivo* imaging.

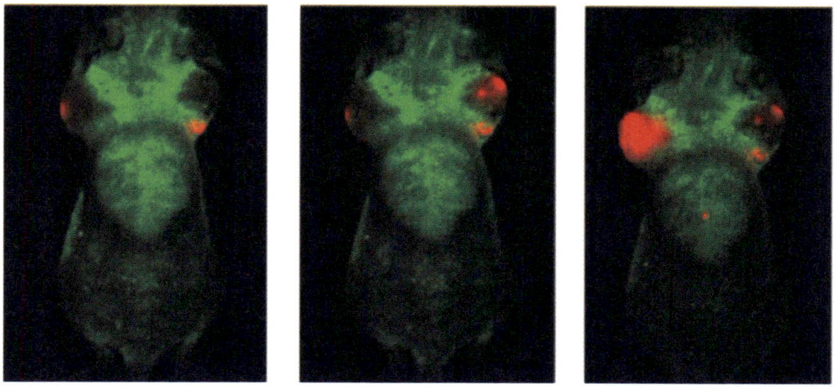

(a) (b) (c)

Fig 4.18. *In vivo* fluorescence images of a Panc-1 tumor-bearing mouse injected intratumorally with the QR/SiO_2 bioconjugate (a) 1, (b) 5 and (c) 10 min post-injection. Reprinted with permission from Ref. [22]. Copyright (2010) American Chemical Society.

If QRs are incorporated with other materials with an imaging function, the resulting nanocomposites can possess multimodal imaging properties. For example, nanocomposites containing QRs and magnetic nanoparticles may be suitable for both fluorescence and magnetic resonance (MR) imaging, while nanocomposites consisting of QRs and gold nanoparticles may be useful for fluorescence and photoacoustic imaging or/and computed tomography imaging. Multimodal imaging techniques are important for improving the level of cancer diagnosis.

Very recently, Gao *et al.* [23] synthesized $CdTe_xSe_{1-x}$/ZnS alloy QRs, then coupled them with paramagnetic gadolinium(III) ions (Gd^{3+}) for *in vivo* dual-modal imaging. They synthesized a series of $CdTe_xSe_{1-x}$ QRs with lengths of 10.8 ± 1, 12.0 ± 1, 12.1 ± 1, and 13.3 ± 1 nm, and found that the fluorescence spectra of the QRs shifted from the visible to near-infrared (NIR) region with increasing ratio of tellurium. They coated the $CdTe_xSe_{1-x}$ QRs with a ZnS shell to improve their fluorescence stability. Finally, they used $CdTe_{0.15}Se_{0.85}$/ZnS QRs with NIR fluorescence (maximum emission: ~800 nm) for animal experiments. The $CdTe_{0.15}Se_{0.85}$/ZnS core–shell QRs were transferred into water by ligand exchange. The water-soluble QRs were modified with an azido-derivatized multidentate polymer (N_3-PMAH). Paramagnetic Gd^{3+} has been widely used in clinical applications as a contrast agent in MR imaging. Positively charged Gd^{3+} was easily adsorbed by the negatively charged $CdTe_{0.15}Se_{0.85}/ZnS$ QRs via electrostatic interactions because the water-soluble QRs contained abundant carboxyl groups. The resulting QR/Gd^{3+} particles were then coated with a PEG-dibenzocyclooctyne layer to protect and stabilize the adsorbed Gd^{3+} by steric shielding, as well as to prevent metal-induced colloid aggregation of the QRs. Gao and co-workers then subcutaneously injected the QR/Gd^{3+}/PEG nanocomposite (10 mg/mL, 0.02 mL) into a paw of a healthy mouse for regional lymph node (LN) mapping. Strong NIR fluorescence emitted in the axillary region was observed in real time without surgical management. This bright fluorescence in the axillary region originated from the QR/Gd^{3+}/PEG nanocomposite, which traveled from the injection site through the lymphatic system to migrate to an axillary LN. The fluorescently labeled LN could also be detected by MR imaging. The T1-weighted MR image shows the enhanced MR signal intensity in this LN. These results indicate that the QR/Gd^{3+}/PEG nanocomposite could be used as a dual-modal nanoprobe for *in vivo* imaging including sentinel LN mapping.

6. Discussion

Compared with QDs, the electronic structures and optical properties of QRs not only depend on their size and surface state, but also their aspect ratio [1, 9, 10]. For example, both the Stokes shift and emission wavelength of QRs increase with their length [1, 10, 24]. The surface area of a single semiconductor QR is much larger than that of a single QD. This allows a single QR to conjugate more biomolecules than a single QD. For example, a CdSe/CdS QR with a length of 24.8 ±3.6 nm and width of 8.2 ± 1.3 nm (aspect ratio: ~3.1 ± 0.5) has a surface area of about 750 mm^2, which is sufficient area for about 42 firefly luciferase molecules to attach to its surface. However, when the aspect ratio of the QR is decreased to 1.8, its surface area decreases to about 216 mm^2 and only 12 luciferase molecules can attach to its surface [25]. The most attractive properties of QRs may be that they are brighter fluorescent probes with slower decay rates than QDs. As a result, a small amount of QRs can light up the target cells or tissues by their strong fluorescence for a long time. For example, when PEG-functionalized CdSe/CdS QRs were injected into the left adductor muscles of living mice (10 μL, 0.025 nmol for each mouse), fluorescence from the QRs was observed 21 days after injection, whereas little fluorescence was detected from equivalent QDs [26].

Although QRs possess excellent optical properties for biomedical imaging, fluorescence imaging has several disadvantages, such as strong background autofluorescence and the limited ability of excitation and emission light to penetrate animal tissues. To overcome these limitations, Alam *et al.* [25] modified CdSe/CdS and CdSe/CdS/ZnS QRs with firefly luciferase from *Photinus pyralis* and found that QRs conjugated with the firefly pyralis luciferase variant PpyGRTS exhibited high bioluminescence resonance energy transfer (BRET) ratios. Because QR fluorescence could be excited by the luminescence of luciferase molecules adsorbed on the QR surface in the presence of the substrate firefly luciferin, no external excitation was needed for the biomedical imaging. Importantly, the efficiency of BRET in this QR system was higher than that of the corresponding QD system. Approaches using BRET may improve the properties of QR systems for *in vivo* biomedical imaging.

Interestingly, hematoxylin and eosin staining of the tissue sections obtained from the mice injected with PEG-coated CdSe/CdS QRs did not show invasion by inflammatory cells 3, 7 or 21 days after intramuscular injection (10 μL, 0.025 nmol for each mouse). In addition, CdSe/CdS QRs were less toxic to cells than CdSe/ZnS QDs [12]. However, both QRs and QDs are very small nanocrystals that readily penetrate animal tissues. It seems reasonable that the strong ability of inorganic nanoparticles to penetrate tissues may also increase their toxicity because these small inorganic nanomaterials can penetrate across several important physiological barriers such as blood–placenta barrier and blood–milk barrier. Both QRs and QDs contain heavy metal ions, and in particular, Cd ions are notably toxic. It is known that the toxicity of QRs and QDs depends on dose. Large animals or humans may require a larger dose of QRs and QDs than smaller animals, and the long-term toxicity of such materials is not clear. Therefore, low-toxicity Cd-free QRs should be developed in the future.

References

[1] Peng X, Manna L, Yang W, Wickham J, Scher E, Kadavanich A and Alivisatos AP. (2000). Shape control of CdSe nanocrystals. *Nature*, **404**:59–61.

[2] Peng ZA and Peng X. (2001). Formation of high-quality CdTe, CdSe, and CdS nanocrystals using CdO as precursor. *J. Am. Chem. Soc.*, **123**:183–184.

[3] Chen CC, Chao CY and Lang ZH. (2000). Simple solution-phase synthesis of soluble CdS and CdSe nanorods. *Chem. Mater.*, **12**:1516.

[4] Panda AB, Glaspell G and El-Shall MS. (2006). Microwave synthesis of highly aligned ultra narrow semiconductor rods and wires. *J. Am. Chem. Soc.*, **128**:2790–2791.

[5] Wang F and Buhro WE. (2007). Determination of the rod-wire transition length in colloidal indium phosphide quantum rods. *J. Am. Chem. Soc.*, **129**:14381–14387.

[6] Shweky I, Aharoni A, Mokari T, Rothenberg E, Nadler M, Podov I and Banin U. (2006). Seeded growth of InP and InAs quantum rods using indium acetate and myristic acid. *Materials Science & Engineering C-Biomimetic And Supramolecular Systems*, **26**:788–794.

[7] Carbone L, Nobile C, De Giorgi M, Sala FD, Morello G, Pompa P, Hytch M, Snoeck E, Fiore A, Franchini IR, Nadasan M, Silvestre AF, Chiodo L, Kudera S, Cingolani R, Krahne R and Manna l. (2007). Synthesis and micrometer-scale assembly of colloidal CdSe/CdS nanorods prepared by a seeded growth approach. *Nano. Lett.*, **7**:2942–2950.

[8] Jacob JM, Balakrishnan RM and Kumar UB. (2014). Biosynthesis of lead selenide quantum rods in marine Aspergillus terreus. *Mater. Lett.*, **124**: 279–281.

[9] Talaat H, Abdallah T, Mohamed MB, Negm S and El-Sayed MA. (2009). The sensitivity of the energy band gap to changes in the dimensions of the CdSe quantum rods at room temperature: STM and theoretical studies. *Chem. Phys. Lett.*, **473**:288–292.

[10] Shieh F, Saunders AE and Korgel BA. (2005). General shape control of colloidal CdS, CdSe, CdTe quantum rods and quantum rod heterostructures. *J. Phys. Chem. B*. **109**:8538–8542.

[11] Fu AH, Gu WW, Boussert B, Koski K, Gerion D, Manna L, Le Gros M, Larabell CA and Alivisatos AP. (2007). Semiconductor quantum rods as single molecule fluorescent biological labels. *Nano. Lett.*, **7**:179–182.

[12] Deka S, Quarta A, Lupo MG, Falqui A, Boninelli S, Giannini C, Morello G, De Giorgi M, Lanzani G, Spinella C, Cingolani R, Pellergrino T and Manna L. (2009). CdSe/CdS/ZnS double shell nanorods with high photoluminescence efficiency and their exploitation as biolabeling probes. *J. Am. Chem. Soc.*, **131**:2948–2958.

[13] Htoon H, Hollingworth JA, Malko AV, Dickerson R and Klimov VI. (2003). Light amplification in semiconductor nanocrystals: quantum rods versus quantum dots. *Appl. Phys. Lett.*, **82**:4776–4778.

[14] Shabaev A and Efros AL. (2004). 1D exciton spectroscopy of semiconductor nanorods. *Nano Lett.*, **4**:1821–1825.

[15] Hu JT, Li LS, Yang WD, Manna L, Wang LW and Alivisatos AP. (2001). Linearly polarized emission from colloidal semiconductor quantum rods. *Science*, **292**:2060–2063.

[16] Rothenberg E, Kazes M, Shaviv E and Banin U. (2005). Electric field induced switching of the fluorescence of single semiconductor quantum rods. *Nano Lett.*, **5**:1581–1586.

[17] Yong KT, Qian J, Roy I, Lee HH, Bergey EJ, Tramposch KM, He S, Swihart MT, Maitra A and Prasad PN. (2007). Quantum rod bioconjugates as targeted probes for confocal and two-photon fluorescence imaging of cancer cells. *Nano. Lett.*, **7**:761–765.

[18] Yong KT, Roy I, Pudavar HE, Bergey EJ, Tramposch KM, Swihart MT and Prasad PN. (2008). Multiplex imaging of pancreatic cancer cells by using functionalized quantum rods. *Adv. Mater.*, **20**:1412–1417.

[19] Chen Y and Liu LH. (2012). Modern methods for delivery of drugs across the blood-brain barrier. *Adv. Drug. Deliv. Rev.*, **64**:640–665.

[20] Xu G, Yong KT, Roy I, Mahajan SD, Ding H, Schwartz SA and Prasad PN. (2008). Bioconjugated quantum rods as targeted probes for efficient transmigration across an *in vitro* blood-brain barrier. *Bioconjug. Chem.*, **19**:1179–1185.

[21] Yong KT, Hu R, Roy I, Ding H, Vathy LA, Bergey EJ, Mizuma M, Maitra A and Prasad PN. (2009). Tumor targeting and imaging in live animals with functionalized semiconductor quantum rods. *ACS Appl. Mat. Interfaces*, **1**:710–719.

[22] Kumar R, Ding H, Hu R, Yong KT, Roy I, Bergey EJ and Prasad PN. (2010). *In vitro* and *In vivo* optical imaging using water-dispersible, noncytotoxic, luminescent, silica-coated quantum rods. *Chem. Mater.*, **22**:2261–2267.

[23] Gao DY, Zhang PF, Sheng ZH, Hu DH, Gong P, Chen C, Wan Q, Gao G and Cai L. (2014). Highly bright and compact alloyed quantum rods with near infrared emitting: a potential multifunctional nanoplatform for multimodal imaging *in vivo*. *Adv. Funct. Mater.*, **24**:3897–3905.

[24] Chen X, Nazzal AY, Xiao M, Peng ZA and Peng XG. (2002). Photoluminescence from single CdSe quantum rods. *J. Lumin.*, **97**: 205–211.

[25] Alam R, Fontaine DM, Branchini BR and Maye MM. (2012). Designing quantum rods for optimized energy transfer with firefly luciferase enzymes. *Nano Lett.*, **12**:3251–3256.

[26] Zacheo A, Quarta A, Mangoni A, Pompa PP, Mastria R, Capogrossi MC, Rinaldi R and Pellegrino T. (2011). CdSe/CdS semiconductor quantum rods as robust fluorescent probes for paraffin-embedded tissue imaging. *IEEE Trans. Nanobiosci.*, **10**:209–215.

Chapter 5

Semiconductor Quantum Dots for Photodynamic Cancer Therapy

Photodynamic therapy (PDT) using photosensitizers is an adjuvant treatment with a long history in clinical practice. Photosensitizers with excellent properties are required to improve the efficacy of PDT. Because most solid tumors grow in deep tissue, the absorption spectra of photosensitizers need to appear in the near-infrared (NIR) region. The optical properties of semiconductor quantum dots (QDs) depend directly on their size. The absorption spectrum of QDs can be shifted to the red or NIR region by increasing their size. Therefore, QDs may be a good choice for deep-tissue PDT. In addition, upon red or NIR laser irradiation, QDs not only efficiently generate reactive oxygen species (ROS), e.g., singlet oxygen, but also release toxic ions, especially heavy metal cations. Both ROS and heavy metal ions can damage DNA and induce cell apoptosis. In this chapter, the mechanism of QDs in PDT, the PDT behaviors of QDs including those of QDs used directly for cancer PDT, fluorescence resonance energy transfers (FRET)-based PDT and bioluminescence resonance energy transfer (BRET)-based PDT are discussed. The future prospects of QDs in PDT are also considered.

1. Introduction

Thousands of years ago, people in ancient Egypt, India, and China used sunlight as a therapeutic agent to treat a variety of skin diseases [1, 2]. In the 18th and 19th centuries in France, sunlight was also used to treat other diseases besides those of the skin, such as tuberculosis, rickets, and scurvy [3]. People at that time realized that phototherapy using sunlight is a simple and effective method to treat some diseases. One hundred years ago, Danish physician Niels Finsen used red light to successfully treat smallpox and further developed a novel phototherapy — the use of ultraviolet (UV) light generated by a carbon arc for cutaneous tuberculosis treatment [3, 4]. Finsen was awarded a Nobel Prize in 1903 for his great contribution to phototherapy.

Use of photosensitive agents in phototherapy improved its efficacy and yielded the novel therapy termed photodynamic therapy (PDT). One hundred years ago, Raab and von Tappeiner first observed the interesting effect of PDT in living cells [3]. They showed that certain dyes such as acridine orange and eosin irradiated by a light could cause cell death. In 1977, Dougherty *et al.* [5] first used PDT to treat malignant tumors. PDT has now been widely accepted as a therapeutic modality, and it is used either alone or in combination with other treatment methods such as chemotherapy and radiotherapy.

Photosensitizers used in PDT include porphyrins and nonporphyrin compounds [6]. The first photosensitizer approved for clinical use in 1993 was PhotofrinR, which is a porphyrin-based drug. Nonporphyrin photosensitizers include hypericin, methylene blue, cyanine and rhodacyanine dyes and nanomaterials like semiconductor QDs and graphene QDs [7], etc. In this chapter, only the current knowledge on the use of semiconductor QDs in PDT is discussed.

2. Mechanism of PDT

PDT uses photosensitizers that undergo photochemical reactions upon irradiation with a light (e.g., laser) of suitable wavelength to treat local diseases. Therefore, PDT involves two steps; the first is the delivery of photosensitizer to the target site (e.g., tumor). The second step involves irradiation of the target tissue containing the photosensitizer with a light to induce photochemical reactions [8].

The mechanisms involved in PDT are shown in Fig. 5.1 and described as follows [9, 10]: when a photosensitizer is excited with a light of suitable wavelength, the photosensitizer is converted from its

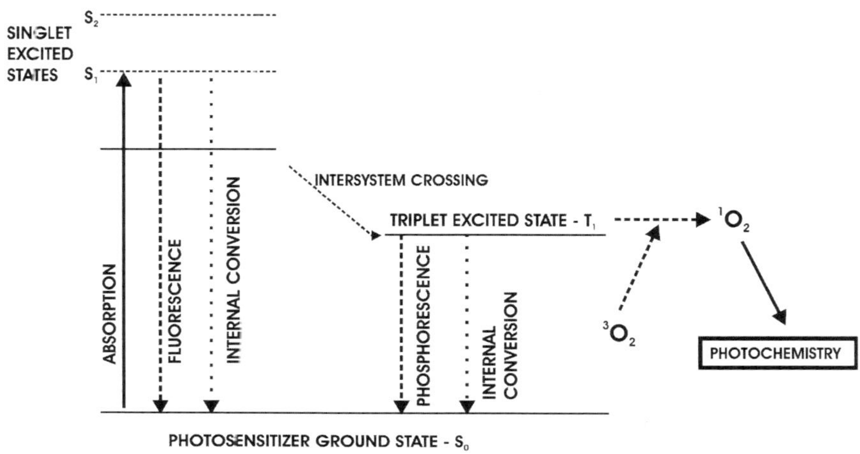

Fig. 5.1. Schematic representation of the photophysical and photochemical processes of PDT. Reprinted with permission from Ref. [9]. Copyright (2006) Elsevier.

stable ground electronic singlet state (S_0) to a short-lived first excited singlet state (S_1). S_1 decays to S_0 by emitting fluorescence or by internal conversion and heat loss. Electrons in S_1 may also be activated to the long-lived triplet excited state (T_1) via intersystem crossing. Photosensitizers in T_1 can react directly with the cell membrane, DNA or other substrate, and transfer protons or electrons to form radicals. These radicals may then react with water to produce ROS including superoxide, hydrogen peroxide, hydroxyl and hydroperoxyl radicals. ROS damage DNA, proteins, specific enzymes, and lipids, which will induce cell death. Photosensitizers in T_1 can also transfer energy to triplet oxygen ($^3O_2$) to produce singlet oxygen ($^1O_2$). $^1O_2$ is very reactive and extremely toxic to cells because it induces biomembrane oxidation and degradation.

The diffusion distance of $^1O_2$ inside a cell is only 10–55 nm [8]; therefore, *in vivo* targeted delivery of photosensitizers is very important for efficacious PDT. For example, photosensitizers should bind specifically to mitochondria, lysosomes or the endoplasmic reticulum to trigger cell death via apoptosis. Conversely, for cancer therapy, only tumor tissue will be irradiated by an excitation light, so only the cancer cells in tumor tissue containing the photosensitizer will be specifically destroyed. This results in minimal damage to the normal tissues surrounding the tumor. In addition, PDT kills cancer cells *in vivo* without causing fibrosis or scarring, unlike surgery and ionizing radiation [8].

The properties of the photosensitizers strongly affect their efficacy in PDT. A large number of photosensitizers have been investigated in the laboratory but only a very small number of photosensitizers are used clinically. An ideal photosensitizer should possess the following eight characteristics [11]: it should (1) have a constant composition, (2) be simple to synthesize and easily available, (3) be nontoxic in the absence of light, (4) exhibit target specificity, (5) possess an excited state with energy higher than 94 kJ/mol (0.97 eV, energy of $^1O_2$), (6) be quickly cleared from the body, (7) display minimal self-aggregation, and (8) be photostable. Few photosensitizers can satisfy all eight of the criteria described above.

3. Direct Use of QDs in Photodynamic Cancer Therapy

3.1 Mechanism of QDs in PDT

The mechanism of semiconductor QDs in PDT is similar to that described above. To clearly illustrate the photophysical and photochemical processes involved in PDT using QDs, another schematic diagram is shown in Fig. 5.2 [11]. When a QD particle is irradiated with a low-energy photon such as UV, visible (VIS) or near infrared (NIR) light, an electron–hole pair (e^-–h^+) will be generated by the QD. The excited QD acts as a charge donor, reacting with the surrounding molecules (acceptor, labeled "A" in Fig. 5.2). This process will produce ROS including superoxide and hydrogen peroxide. In addition, QDs in T_1 state can react with surrounding molecules, and $^3O_2$ is converted into $^1O_2$ during this process. QDs can also be used as energy donors to excite other photosensitizers for cancer PDT (this will be discussed in detail below in Section 4). Semiconductor QDs contain heavy metals such as cadmium (Cd). The release rate of toxic heavy metal ions from the QDs may be accelerated during light irradiation

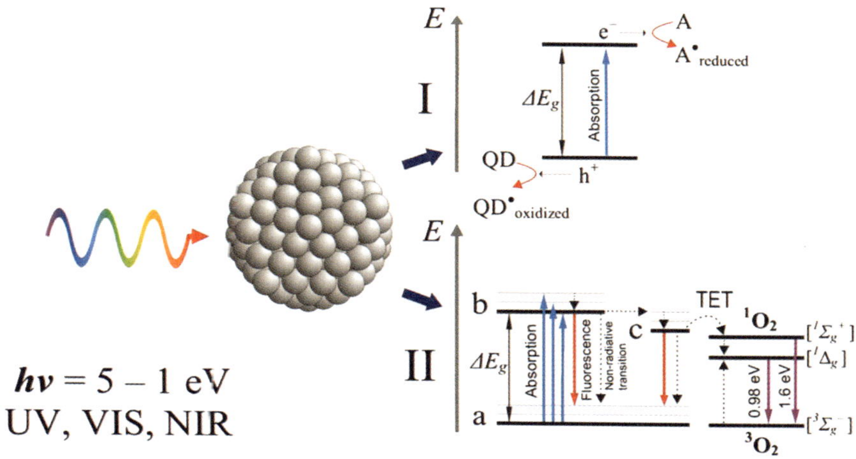

Fig. 5.2. Mechanism of PDT using semiconductor QDs. A is an acceptor molecule. ΔE_g is the energy band-gap of the QD. a, b, and c are the ground state, excited state and "trap" state, respectively. Dashed arrows show nonradiative transitions. TET is triplet energy transfer. Reprinted with permission from Ref. [11]. Copyright (2008) Elsevier.

because of surface oxidation. The ROS and toxic heavy metal ions (e.g., Cd^{2+}) generated by the QDs in tissue or cells after irradiation can kill cancer cells by inducing DNA degradation or damaging other biomolecules. A cancer cell being killed by QDs excited by irradiation is illustrated in Fig. 5.3 [10].

3.2 QDs as photosensitizers for photodynamic cancer therapy

In 2003, Samia *et al.* [12] found that cadmium selenide (CdSe) QDs could generate $^1O_2$ after irradiation. CdSe QDs with a diameter of 5 nm and fluorescence quantum yield in toluene solution at 488 nm of ~65% were excited with light of 488 nm. The emission spectra and decay kinetics of $^1O_2$ generated by the QDs were detected by laser-flash photolysis and a liquid nitrogen-cooled germanium detector positioned behind a 1200 nm long-pass filter and coupled to a digital oscilloscope. The emission of $^1O_2$

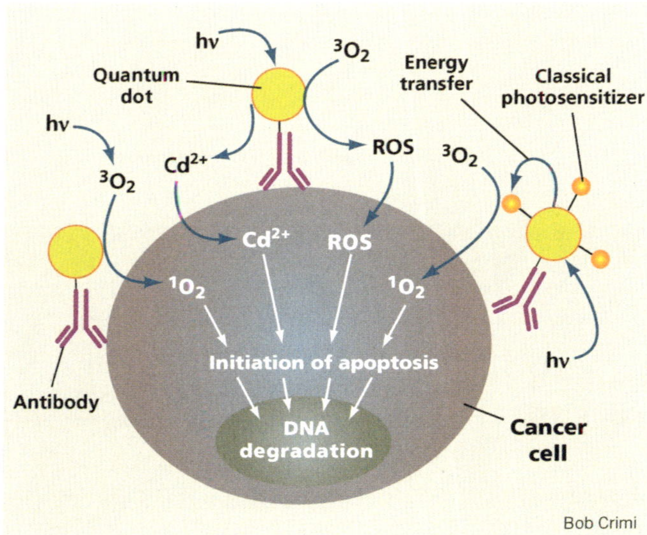

Fig. 5.3. Possible mechanisms of QDs in cancer PDT. Reprinted with permission from Ref. [10]. Copyright (2004) Nature Publishing Group.

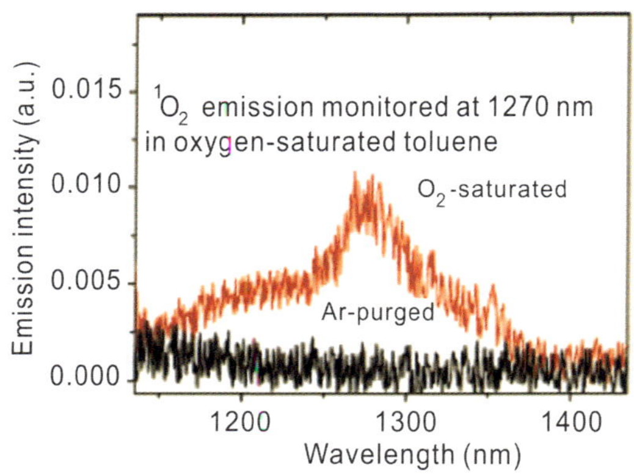

Fig. 5.4. Emission spectra of $^1O_2$ generated from CdSe QDs in toluene solution following excitation at 488 nm. Reprinted with permission from Ref. [12]. Copyright (2003) American Chemical Society.

generated by the QDs was located at 1270 nm (Fig. 5.4), and the $^1O_2$ quantum yield was about 5%. The decay rate of $^1O_2$ emission from the CdSe QDs in oxygen-saturated solution was obviously slower than that of the CdSe QDs in argon-purged solution, which indicated that oxygen played an important role in the production of $^1O_2$.

Bakalova *et al.* [13] demonstrated that CdSe QDs could produce free radicals after UV irradiation. They added water-soluble CdSe QDs into a suspension of unilamellar egg-yolk lecinine liposomes, then irradiated the mixture with UV light of 340 nm. They found that the amount of the end product from the free radical oxidation of polyunsaturated fatty acid residues, malondialdehyde (MDA), increased with the concentration of CdSe QDs after UV irradiation, which indicated that the QDs excited during UV-vis illumination delivered charges to lipids, then produced free radicals. These free radicals reacted with the liposomes. In addition, when iron(II) ions (Fe^{2+}) and ascorbate were added to the suspension of CdSe QDs and liposomes to induce lipid peroxidation in the liposomes, more MDA was produced after irradiation, and the yield of MDA increased more rapidly with increasing QD concentration than that in the system without Fe^{2+} and ascorbate. These radicals as well as the ROS generated by the CdSe QDs upon UV-vis illumination can effectively damage cancer cells. To specifically kill cancer cells, Bakalova *et al.* conjugated anti-CD90 antibody onto water-soluble CdSe QDs. The anti-CD90-conjugated QDs were then incubated with leukemia cells or a mixture of leukemia cells and normal lymphocytes. After the cells were irradiated with UV light of 340 nm for 1 h (three cycles of 10 min with and 10 min without irradiation), only the leukemia cells were seriously damaged; the viability of the normal lymphocytes did not markedly decrease.

To investigate whether DNA molecules could be damaged by semiconductor QDs upon photoactivation, in 2008, Anas *et al.* [14] prepared plasmid DNA (pDNA)-QD bioconjugates by reacting biotinylated pDNA with streptavidin-functionalized CdSe/zinc sulfide (ZnS) QDs. They then investigated the photosensitized breakage of strands and nucleobase damage in the pDNA-QD conjugates after exposure to a laser beam in the presence of oxygen. As shown in Fig. 5.5a, when the pDNA-QD conjugates were irradiated with 400 nm light with an intensity of 1 W/cm^2 for 1 h, agarose gel electrophoresis images revealed a decrease in the intensity of the supercoiled conformer of the photoactivated pDNA-QD conjugates compared with that of the unactivated ones. Meanwhile, the image of the pDNA-QD conjugates kept in the dark for 1 h was similar to

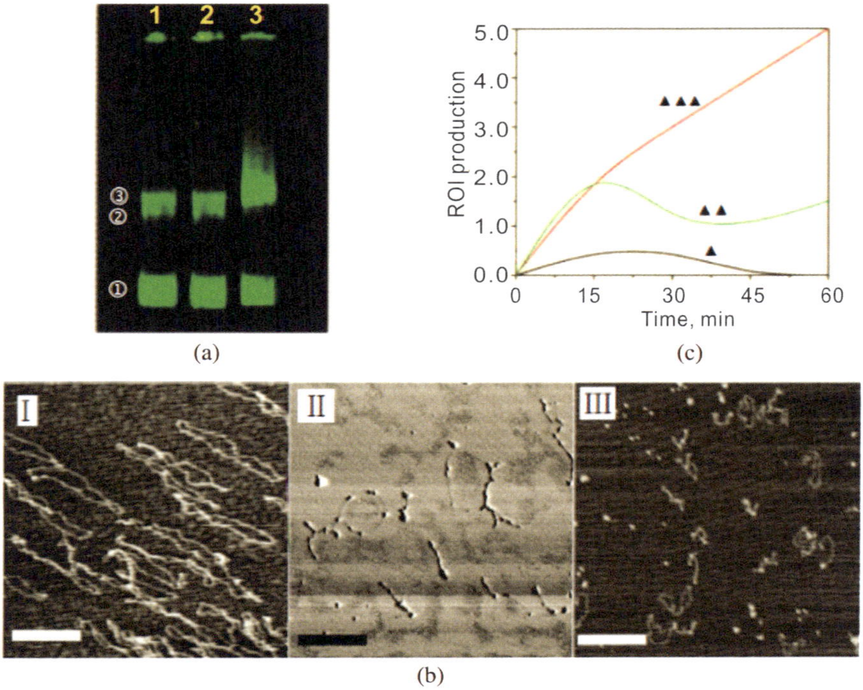

Fig. 5.5. (a) Agarose gel electrophoresis images of pDNA-QD conjugates: (lane 1) freshly prepared sample, (lane 2) incubated in the dark for 1 h, and (lane 3) photoactivated at 400 nm for 1 h. ① Supercoiled, ② circular, and ③ linear conformers of pDNA. (b) AFM images of (I) biotinylated pDNA, (II) pDNA-QD conjugates prepared by reacting pDNA with ~20 biotin units with QDs, (III) pDNA-QD conjugates irradiated with 532 nm light for 1 h (the biotinylated pDNA had ~20 biotin moieties). The scale bars are 800, 600, and 500 nm in (I), (II) and (III), respectively. (c) Nitroblue tetrazolium (NBT) assay of reactive oxygen intermediate (ROI) production by QDs (photoluminescence maxima: ~600 nm). Temporal evolution of the optical density at 650 nm of NBT-QD mixtures (▲) incubated in the dark, (▲▲) photoactivated (0.1 W/cm^2 at 532 nm) after purging with nitrogen gas, and (▲▲▲) photoactivated (0.1 W/cm^2 at 532 nm) in the presence of oxygen. Reprinted with permission from Ref. [14]. Copyright (2008) American Chemical Society.

that of the fresh pDNA-QD conjugates (Fig. 5.5a). These results imply that the supercoiled conformer of pDNA in the photoactivated pDNA-QD conjugates was destroyed upon UV irradiation, including the strand breakages and nucleobase damage. Atomic force microscopy (AFM) images further demonstrated that the supercoiled conformer of pDNA was damaged by the photosensitized reactions with QDs. As shown in Fig. 5.5b, when pDNA-QD conjugates with a low density of QDs (<20 QDs/pDNA) were irradiated with 532 nm light with an intensity of 1 W/cm^2 for 1 h, fragments of the pDNA-QD conjugate were clearly observed. The pDNA in the equivalent pDNA-QD conjugates that were not irradiated retained their normal circular supercoiled structure (Fig. 5.5b). The photosensitized strand breakage and nucleobase damage in the pDNA were mainly caused by the reaction of the pDNA with ROS produced by the photoactivated QDs, because QDs photoactivated in the presence of oxygen readily produce reactive oxygen intermediates over time (Fig. 5.5c).

Our research group found that cadmium telluride (CdTe) and copper indium sulfide ($CuInS_2$)/ZnS QDs in aqueous solution could produce high levels of intracellular ROS after 671-nm laser irradiation [15, 16]. For example, when human A375 melanoma cells were incubated with CdTe QDs with an emission maxima of 710 nm and concentration of only 0.05 mg/mL, and then irradiated with a 671-nm laser (0.2 W/cm^2) for 20 min, the ROS level in the A375 cells was 5.28 ± 2.14 times higher than that in the control experiment (nonirradiated cells in the absence of QDs) [15].

4. Quantum Dots for Photodynamic Cancer Therapy based on Resonance Energy Transfer

In Chapter 3, we discussed QD systems that operate through bioluminescence resonance energy transfer (BRET). Resonance energy transfer techniques include not only BRET, but also fluorescence resonance energy transfer (FRET). Both of these processes involve nonradiative energy transfer from a donor molecule or nanoparticle to an energy acceptor located near the donor. Just like BRET, FRET also has two important requirements: the first is that the fluorescent emission spectrum of the donor and the absorption spectrum of the acceptor should have a large overlap, and the second is that the distance between the donor and acceptor should not exceed 10 nm [17]. Unlike BRET, FRET does require an external excitation light. Cancer PDT based on BRET or FRET with QDs as the energy donor is an interesting approach that has attracted considerable attention recently.

4.1 BRET-based PDT using QDs as energy acceptors and donors

As mentioned above, photosensitizers for PDT need to be excited with an external light of a suitable wavelength. For *in vivo* cancer therapy, the wavelength of this external excitation light should be in the near-infrared (NIR) band. Although the ability of NIR light to penetrate tissues is much higher than that of light of shorter wavelength, the depth that NIR light can penetrate is still limited, which results in less ROS being generated by photosensitizers trapped in deep tissue, and thus in lower PDT efficacy. To overcome this limitation, in 2013, Hsu *et al.* [18] employed bioluminescent QDs as an internal light source for BRET-based PDT using meta-tetra-hydroxyphenyl-chlorin (m-THPC) as a photosensitizer. A QD-BRET system was first developed by So and co-workers in 2006 [19]. In their system, the enzyme renilla luciferase 8 (Luc8) coated on the QD surface was an important energy donor. When the QD-Luc8 conjugates were reacted with the substrate coelenterazine, strong bioluminescence at about 480 nm emitted by the Luc8 shell was absorbed by the QD core, which then emitted red or NIR fluorescence.

Such QD-Luc8 conjugates can also be used as an energy donor to activate specific photosensitizers for cancer PDT. To ensure highly efficacious cancer PDT, the QD-Luc8 conjugate should be near the photosensitizer, the *in vivo* activity of Luc8 and coelenterazine should be high, and the Luc8 molecules coated on the QD surface should not be easily released from the QDs *in vivo*. Hsu *et al.* [18] used QDs with an emission wavelength of 655 nm for BRET-based PDT in a mouse model. As shown in Fig. 5.6, the red fluorescence emitted by QD-Luc8 conjugates could be used to excite nearby photosensitizers. When this QD-Luc8/photosensitizer system was used for PDT, only coelenterazine needed to be added; excitation with external light was not required. Therefore, tumors in deep tissue may be treated by this kind of PDT. To investigate whether BRET-based PDT using QD-Luc8 conjugates could be used for *in vivo* cancer therapy, Hsu's group injected a QD-Luc8 conjugate and m-THPC photosensitizer into the tumors of mice with lung cancer grown from A549 cancer cells, then injected coelenterazine into the tail veins of the same mice. Their results showed that the growth of tumors was inhibited from day 3 to 20 after

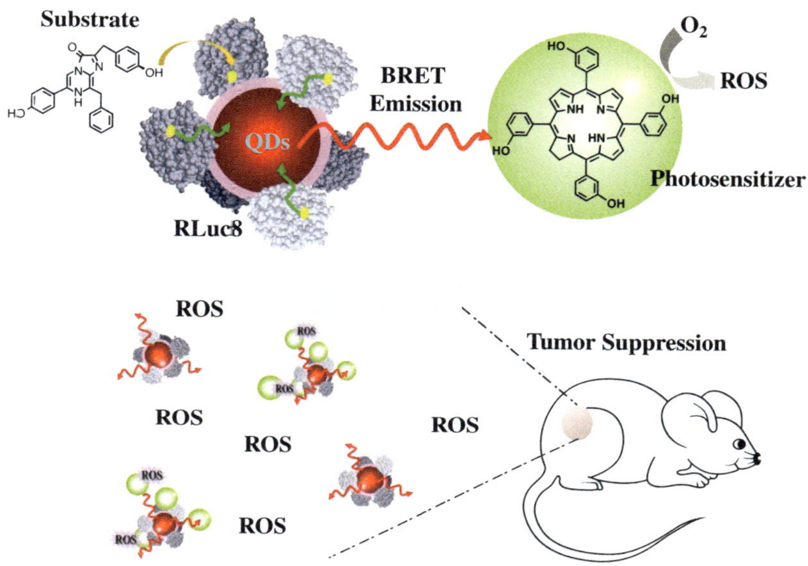

Fig. 5.6. Schematic illustration of BRET-based PDT using Luc8-immobilized QDs. Reprinted with permission from Ref. [18]. Copyright (2012) Elsevier.

treatment compared with that of the control groups. Histologic hematoxylin and eosin-stained tissue sections showed that the cancer cells were damaged and prominent apoptosis was clearly observed in the BRET-based PDT group, whereas almost no damage was detected in the control groups. However, this method may be expensive, and cancer therapy efficiency may be not very high.

4.2 FRET-based PDT using QDs as energy donors

When a fluorescent material excited by external light (not bioluminescence) behaves as an energy donor, and transfers energy nonradiatively to an acceptor material (e.g., photosensitizer) near the donor material, this photophysical process is called FRET. In 2003, Samia *et al.* [12] reported that they had used QD-based FRET to excite a PDT photosensitizer. They conjugated CdSe QDs with a diameter of ~5 nm onto the silicon phthalocyanine 4 (Pc4) photosensitizer through an alkyl amino group on the photosensitizer. When the QD-Pc4 conjugates were irradiated with 488 nm light, the CdSe QDs emitted bright fluorescence ranging from about 500 to 630 nm, and the Pc4 photosensitizer was activated by the QD emission at 568 nm. Although the CdSe QDs themselves could produce ROS after irradiation, the quantum yield of $^1O_2$ was only about 5%, whereas that of the Pc4 photosensitizer was 43%.

QD-photosensitizer conjugates generate $^1O_2$ through FRET or possibly through both FRET and direct external excitation of the photosensitizer. The quantum yield of $^1O_2$ of specific photosensitizers being improved by the addition of QDs was demonstrated by Tekdas and coworkers in 2012 [20]. They synthesized thioglycolic acid (TGA)-capped CdTe QDs with a diameter of 4–5 nm and then mixed the QDs with tetratriethyleneoxythia-substituted aluminum, gallium and indium phthalocyanines (MPc) in dimethyl sulfoxide (DMSO). The fluorescent emission spectrum of the QDs overlapped well with the absorption spectrum of each MPc. For example, the fluorescence of the TGA-CdTe QDs ranged from 500 to 750 nm, while the absorption spectrum of gallium phthalocyanine (GaPc) ranged from 550 to 750 nm (Fig. 5.7a). The MPcs were not chemically linked to the surface of the QDs, but were probably physically adsorbed onto the surface of the QDs. As shown in Fig. 5.7b, GaPc excited by 500 nm light only exhibited low emission intensity ranging from about

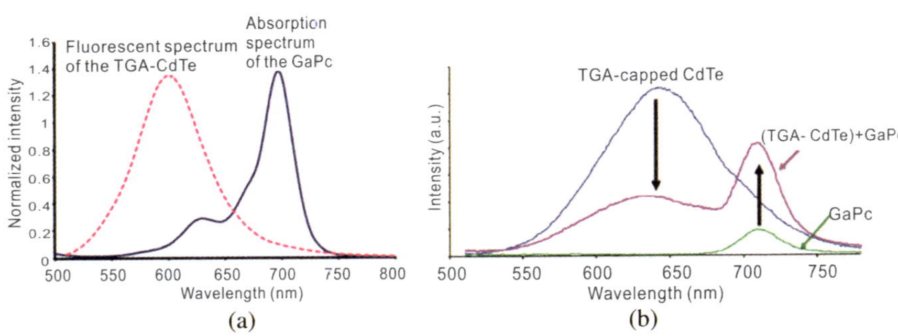

Fig. 5.7. (a) Normalized fluorescent emission spectrum of TGA-capped CdTe QDs (excitation: 500 nm) and absorption spectrum of GaPc. (b) Fluorescent emission spectra (excitation: 500 nm) of the TGA-capped CdTe QDs, GaPc and a mixture of TGA-CdTe and GaPc. Reprinted with permission from Ref. [20]. Copyright (2012) Elsevier.

680 to 750 nm. However, this emission was obviously enhanced after the addition of CdTe QDs. This indicates that the GaPc photosensitizer was excited by QD fluorescence. Importantly, they found that the $^1O_2$ quantum yields of the MPcs were improved when they were mixed with the CdTe QDs. For example, the $^1O_2$ quantum yield of aluminum phthalocyanine (AlPc) in DMSO was 29%, whereas that of a mixture of AlPc and CdTe QDs was 46%. In addition, the presence of QDs increased the stability of the photosensitizers by decreasing MPc photodegradation. Higher $^1O_2$ quantum yield and higher photostability of a photosensitizer are beneficial for cancer PDT. Therefore, the efficacy of FRET-based PDT using QDs as an energy donor may be higher than PDT using the photosensitizer or QDs alone.

In the work by Tekdas' group described above [20], MPc photosensitizers were simply mixed with CdTe QDs. However, the QD-photosensitizer composites formed by such nonspecific attachment do not always exhibit energy transfer because such adsorption may result in a large distance between the QDs and photosensitizers. For example, when positively charged photosensitizer rose bengal (RB) was incubated with negatively charged CdSe/cadmium sulfide (CdS)/ZnS QDs, the resulting QD-RB complexes did not show FRET [21]. Therefore, other researchers have used covalent binding to fabricate QD-photosensitizer composites [21, 22].

However, the QD-photosensitizer conjugates formed by covalent reaction reported to date do not generate more $^1O_2$ than the free photosensitizers. For example, Tsay *et al.* [21] conjugated RB and chlorin e6 (Ce6) to CdSe/CdS/ZnS QDs with emission maxima of 538 and 620 nm, respectively, through covalent bonding. To protect the photophysical properties of both the QDs and photosensitizers, the photosensitizers were conjugated with peptides, then reacted with the peptide-coated QDs (Fig. 5.8). One QD could be conjugated with up to 30 photosensitizer molecules by this method. When the QD-RB and QD-Ce6 conjugates were excited by light of 450 nm, the intensities of fluorescence from both RB and Ce6 in the conjugates dramatically increased compared with those of the same concentrations of unconjugated RB and Ce6 (Fig. 5.9). This implies that FRET occurred between the QDs and photosensitizers. However, the $^1O_2$ quantum yields of QD-RB and QD-Ce6 were 17% and 31%, respectively, which were lower than those of the unconjugated photosensitizers. This

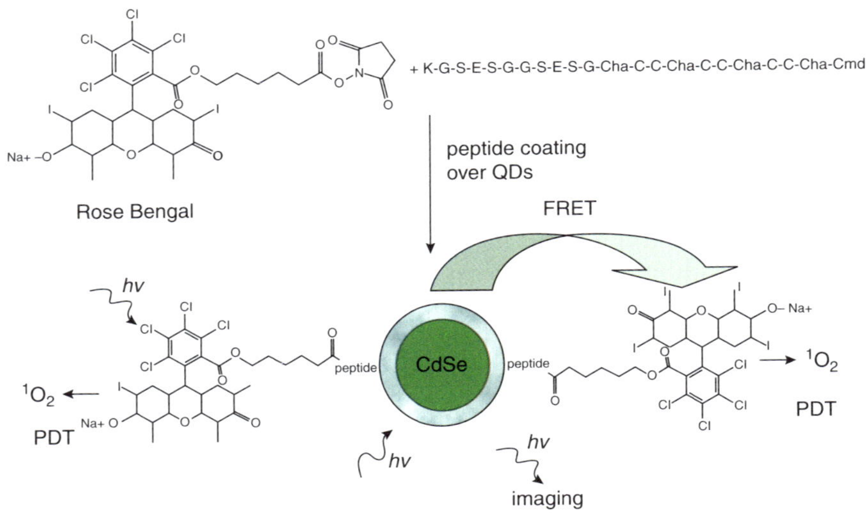

Fig. 5.8. Schematic illustration of the conjugation of RB photosensitizer to CdSe/CdS/ZnS QDs and ${}^1O_2$ generation based on FRET. QD-Ce6 was formed in a similar manner to QD-RB. Reprinted with permission from Ref. [21]. Copyright (2007) American Chemical Society.

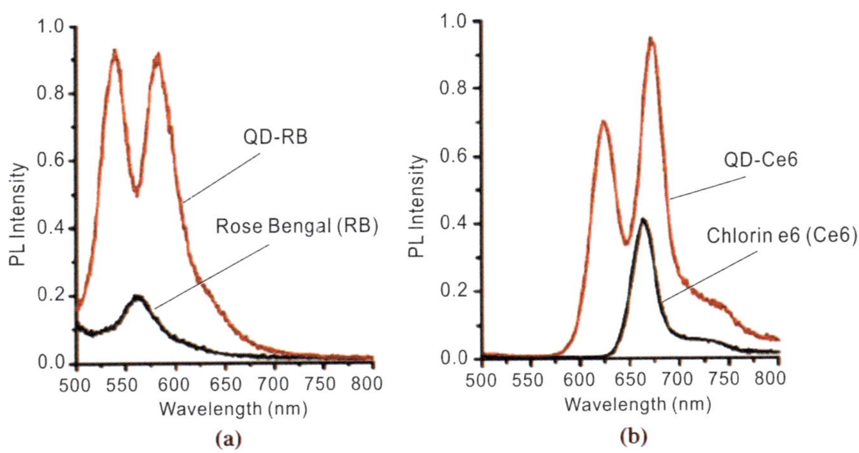

Fig. 5.9. Photoluminescence (PL) emission spectra. (a) RB-conjugated CdSe/CdS/ZnS QDs with an emission maxima of 538 nm and an equal concentration of RB excited at 450 nm. (b) Ce6-conjugated QDs with an emission maxima of 620 nm and an equal concentration of Ce6 alone excited at 450 nm. Reprinted with permission from Ref. [21]. Copyright (2007) American Chemical Society.

indicates that the efficacy of FRET is low because the QDs still exhibit strong fluorescence. However, these QD-photosensitizer composites may still be useful for cancer PDT based on FRET, and as fluorescent probes for biomedical imaging.

In 2012, Charron *et al.* [22] synthesized silica-coated indium phosphide (InP)/ZnS QDs and then conjugated Ce6 photosensitizer onto the QDs via covalent reaction. The resulting InP/ZnS QD-Ce6 nanocomposite may exhibit lower toxicity than the Cd-based systems described above. The energy transfer pathways of the QD-Ce6 nanocomposite are illustrated in Fig. 5.10. The $^1O_2$ quantum yield of InP/ZnS QD-Ce6 excited by UV light of 350 nm was slightly lower than that of free Ce6. In addition, when breast carcinoma MDA-MB-231 cells were incubated with InP/ZnS QD-Ce6 or a similar concentration of free Ce6, then irradiated with 350 nm UV light for 5 min, the cell viabilities of these two groups were similar (~60%) (Fig. 5.11). To improve the efficacy of PDT,

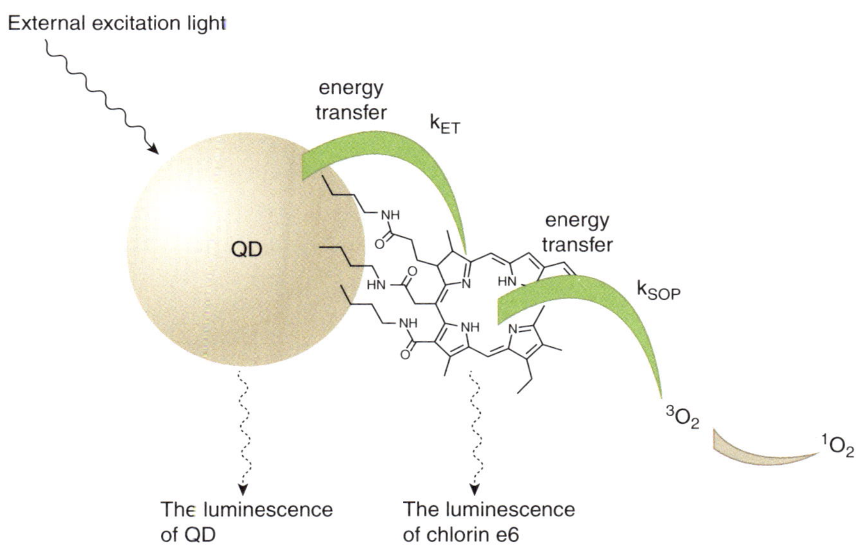

Fig. 5.10. Energy transfer pathways in QD/Ce6 hybrids. k_{ET} denotes the rate constant for energy transfer from the QDs to Ce6, while k_{SOP} is that for energy transfer from Ce6 to oxygen. Reprinted with permission from Ref. [22]. Copyright (2012) American Chemical Society.

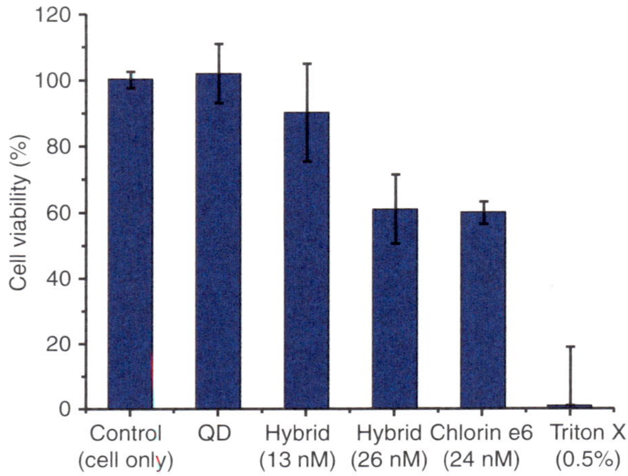

Fig. 5.11. Viabilities of MDA-MB-231 cancer cells incubated with InP/ZnS QDs, Ce6 or QD-Ce6 hybrid for 3 h then irradiated with UV light (0.033 J/cm^2) for 5 min. Reprinted with permission from Ref. [22]. Copyright (2012) American Chemical Society.

the efficacy of FRET between the QDs and photosensitizer should be increased. The efficacy of FRET may be tuned by choosing QD donors and photosensitizer acceptors with an appropriate degree of spectral overlap and by changing the distance between the QD and photosensitizer [20]. Therefore, the efficacy of FRET may be improved by adjusting the optical properties of the QDs, the size of linker molecules between the QDs and photosensitizer, or the method used to conjugate the photosensitizer with QDs.

5. Discussion

As mentioned above, QDs can be directly used as photosensitizers for cancer PDT. QDs can also act as an energy acceptor or donor for BRET- or FRET-based PDT. In addition, the metal ions released from QDs during irradiation help to fight cancer cells. Therefore, QDs may be good reagents for cancer PDT. In QD-BRET systems, the bioactivity of luciferase conjugated on the QD surface and amount of substrate molecules around the luciferase both decrease over time because of the reaction between the luciferase and substrate. Therefore, QD-BRET systems may not be suitable for long-term PDT.

QDs used for *in vivo* imaging and cancer therapy can be divided into two classes. The first is Cd-containing QDs such as CdTe QDs, and the second is Cd-free QDs like lnP/ZnS QDs. Cd is a probable carcinogen that has a long biological half-life in humans [23]. As a result, Cd-containing QDs may not be suitable for human cancer PDT. The toxicity of Cd-free QDs is obviously lower than that of Cd-containing ones. If Cd-free QDs are protected by a polymer with good biocompatibility or by an inorganic shell (e.g., silica), and if a low dosage of these QDs exhibits highly efficacious cancer therapy, then they might be attractive candidates as photosensitizers for clinical use. Cancer PDT is a local treatment method, and photosensitizers can be intratumorally injected. It has been demonstrated that when QDs were directly injected into a mouse tumor, only a small amount of the QDs and/or metal ions had leaked from the tumor 15 days after injection [15]. Intratumoral injection may reduce the toxicity of QDs to the rest of the body compared with intravenous injection. Therefore, when low-toxicity QDs with appropriate surface protection are injected into a body using a low dosage and an appropriate route of administration, they may have potential for clinical application in cancer PDT.

Semiconductor quantum rods (QRs) can also generate ROS after being irradiated by a laser, so they have potential for use in cancer PDT. Because a single QR has brighter fluorescence than a single QD of the same material (e.g., a CdTe QR and CdTe QD), the efficacy of PDT using a QR-BRET system may be higher than that of the equivalent QD-BRET system. In addition, a QR-FRET system may be more suitable for both fluorescent imaging and PDT than the corresponding QD-FRET system.

References

[1] Spikes JD. (1985). The historical development of ideas on applications of photosensitised reactions in health sciences. In Bergasson G, Jori Land EJ and Truscott TG. *Primary Photoprocesses in Biology and Medicine*. New York. R. V: Plenum Press, 209–227.

[2] Epstein JM. (1990). Phototherapy and photochemotherapy. *N. Engl. J. Med.*, **32**:1149–1151.

[3] Ackroyd R, Kelty C, Brown N and Reed M. (2001). The history of photodetection and photodynamic therapy. *Photochem Photobiol.*, **74**: 656–669.

[4] Finsen NR. (1901). *Phototherapy*. London: Edward Arnold.

[5] Dougherty TJ, Kaufman JE, Goldfarb A, Weishaupt KR, Boyle D and Mittleman A. (1978). Photoradiation therapy for the treatment of malignant tumors. *Cancer Res.*, **38**:2628–2635.

[6] Paszko E, Ehrhardt C, Senge MO, Kelleher DP and Reynolds JV. (2011). Nanodrug applications in photodynamic therapy. *Photodiagnosis Photodyn Ther.*, **8**:14–29.

[7] Shibua ES, Hamadaa M, Murasea N and Biju V. (2013). Nanomaterials formulations for photothermal and photodynamic therapy of cancer. *J. Photochem Photobiol A Chem.*, **15**:53–72.

[8] Anand S, Ortel BJ, Pereira SP, Hasan T and Maytin EV. (2012). Biomodulatory approaches to photodynamic therapy for solid tumors. *Cancer Lett.*, **326**:8–16.

[9] Stylli SS and Kaye AH. (2006). Photodynamic therapy of cerebral glioma — a review. Part II — clinical studies. *J Clin Neurosci.*, **13**:709–717.

[10] Bakalova R, Ohba H, Zhelev Z, Ishikawa M and Baba Y. (2004). Quantum dots as photosensitizers? *Nat. Biotechnol.*, **22**:1360–1361.

[11] Juzenas P, Chen W, Sun YP, Coelho MA, Generalov R, Generalova N and Christensen IL. (2008). Quantum dots and nanoparticles for photodynamic and radiation therapies of cancer. *Adv. Drug Deliv. Rev.*, **60**:1600–1614.

[12] Samia AC, Chen X and Burda C. (2003). Semiconductor quantum dots for photodynamic therapy. *J. Am. Chem. Soc.*, **125**:15736–15737.

[13] Rumiana Bakalova, Hideki Ohba, Zhivko Zhelev, Toshimi Nagase, Rajan Jose,Mitsuru Ishikawa and Yoshinobu Baba. (2004). Quantum dot anti-CD conjugates: are they potential photosensitizers or potentiators of classical photosensitizing agents in photodynamic therapy of cancer? *Nano Lett.*, 4(9):1567–1573.

[14] Anas A, Akita H, Harashima H, Itoh T, Ishikawa M and Biju V. (2008). Photosensitized breakage and damage of DNA by CdSe-ZnS quantum dots. *J. Phys. Chem. B.*, **112**:10005–10011.

[15] Chu M, Pan X, Zhang D, Wu Q, Peng J and Hai W. (2012). The therapeutic efficacy of CdTe and CdSe quantum dots for photothermal cancer therapy. *Biomaterials.*, **33**:7071–7083.

[16] Wu Q, Chu MQ, Shao YX, Wo FJ and Shi DL. (2016). Reduced graphene oxide conjugated with CuInS2/ZnS nanocrystals with low toxicity for enhanced photothermal and photodynamic cancer therapies. *Carbon*, **108**: 21–37.

[17] Milligan G. (2004). Applications of bioluminescence- and fluorescence resonance energy transfer to drug discovery at G protein-coupled receptors. *Eur. J. Pharm Sci.*, **21**:397–405.

[18] Hsu CY, Chen CW, Yu HP, Lin YF and Lai PS. (2013). Bioluminescence resonance energy transfer using luciferase-immobilized quantum dots for self-illuminated photodynamic therapy. *Biomaterials.*, **34**:1204–1212.

[19] So MK, Xu CJ, Loening AM, Gambhir SS and Rao JH. (2006). Self-illuminating quantum dot conjugates for *in vivo* imaging. *Nat. Biotechnol.*, **24**:339–343.

[20] Tekdas DA, Durmus M, Yanik H and Ahsen V. (2012). Photodynamic therapy potential of thiol-stabilized CdTe quantum dot-group 3A phthalocyanine conjugates (QD-Pc). *Spectrochim Acta A Mol. Biomol. Spectrosc.*, **93**:313–320.

[21] Tsay JM, Trzoss M, Shi L, Kong X, Selke M, Jung ME and Weiss S. (2007). Singlet oxygen production by Peptide-coated quantum dot-photosensitizer conjugates. *J. Am. Chem Soc.*, **129**:6865–6871.

[22] Charron G, Stuchinskaya T, Edwards DR, Russell DA and Nann T. (2012). Insights into the mechanism of quantum dot-sensitized singlet oxygen production for photodynamic therapy. *J. Phys. Chem. C.*, **116**:9334–9342.

[23] Jolibois LS, Jr.. Burow ME, Swan KF, George WJ, Anderson MB and Henson MC. (1999). Effects of cadmium cell viability, trophoblastic development, and expression of low density lipoprotein receptor transcripts in cultured human placental cells. *Reprod. Toxicol.*, **13**:473–480.

Chapter 6

Semiconductor Quantum Dots for Photothermal Cancer Therapy

Semiconductor quantum dots (QDs) are novel powerful fluorescent nanoprobes that can be used for *in vitro* and *in vivo* biomedical labeling and imaging. QDs have attracted considerable attention from biomedical researchers during the past decade because they exhibit several unique optical properties compared with conventional fluorescent dyes. Recently, researchers found that QDs can also kill cancer cells through their photothermal effect. QDs with deep colors, such as brown or close to black, are more suitable for *in vivo* cancer photothermal therapy (PTT) than those with light colors like yellow and red. This is because deeply colored QDs strongly absorb in the red and near-infrared (NIR) region. NIR light can penetrate deep into animal tissues, and deeply colored QDs can efficiently convert NIR light into heat energy, which can damage cells. PTT is a new direction of research for QDs. In this chapter, the use of cadmium- and copper-based QDs, for cancer PTT is discussed. The advantages and disadvantages of these QDs in PTT as well as their future prospects in this field are considered.

1. Introduction

Compared with normal tissue, tumor tissue is hypoxic and at lower pH [1]. The cancer cells in this specific environment are more sensitive to high temperature than the cells in normal tissue. It has been demonstrated that cancer cells were killed at temperatures over 42.5°C, whereas normal cells could survive up to 44°C [2, 3]. In addition, the blood flow in tumor tissue is lower than that in normal tissue, which makes the tumor less able to dissipate heat, so the temperature of tumor tissue is increased more easily than that of normal tissue. Therefore, increasing the temperature of a whole body or local region can be used for cancer therapy. Killing cancer cells by heating them has attracted worldwide interest since 1975 [4]. The temperature used in such treatments ranges from hyperthermic (41–48°C) to high-temperature thermal ablation (heating to ~70°C). This type of treatment is called thermal therapy, and has been successfully used in clinical settings.

Two types of hyperthermia methods have been clinically applied: whole-body hyperthermia and partial-body hyperthermia. The latter includes regional and local hyperthermia. For whole-body hyperthermia, the body temperature should be rigorously controlled (usually in the range from 41.8 to 42°C [4]) to avoid negative effects caused by heating the whole body. Regional hyperthermia is used to treat larger parts of the body such as a limb, organ or body cavity. Local hyperthermia usually heats the tumor alone to increase its temperature. Compared with whole-body and regional hyperthermia, local hyperthermia can minimize damage to healthy tissue while the cancer cells are killed. These hyperthermia methods result in protein denaturation, changes in the cytoskeleton, membrane and other multimolecular structures, and weakened DNA synthesis and repair [4, 5]. The efficacy of a thermal treatment depends on the temperature used and exposure time [4].

The heat for local hyperthermia can be generated with microwaves, radio-frequency waves, ultrasound, magnetic hyperthermia under alternating magnetic field, and laser irradiation. Compared with other hyperthermia modalities, Red or NIR laser irradiation is a convenient and low-cost technique that can efficiently induce cancer cell death. The use of laser light-induced hyperthermia/thermal ablation to treat disease including cancer is termed photothermal therapy (PTT) [6].

However, healthy tissues are usually also destroyed during hyperthermia treatment. This is because both healthy and cancerous tissues can absorb the laser light energy. Therefore, in conventional PTT, laser irradiation induces nonspecific damage of the adjacent tissues [6].

Local hyperthermia combined with the use of nanoparticles can overcome this limitation. This is because nanoparticles can efficiently generate heat after being stimulated by external laser light irradiation with low power density. After nanoparticles accumulate in tumor tissue, they can specifically destroy tumor cells following irradiation, avoiding damage to the normal tissues. For example, when polyethylene glycol (PEG)-passivated NIR-absorbing gold nanoshells were injected into a mouse tumor and then exposed to NIR laser light (820 nm, 4 W/cm^2), maximal temperature changes were observed only beneath the apical surface because the nanoshells mainly accumulated at this site [7]. The surrounding tissue near the tumor remained at lower temperature, and the tissue without nanoshells also did not generate much heat after irradiation. Besides highly efficient heat generation, the nanoparticles used for local hyperthermia should also possess the following properties: (1) exhibit low or no toxicity without the external stimulus, (2) be smaller than 100 nm so that they can readily migrate to the tumor, (3) disperse well in aqueous solution, and (4) possess surfaces that can be conveniently conjugated with cell recognition moieties [6].

As mentioned above, combining nanoparticles and laser irradiation with low power density for local cancer therapy is a safe modality compared with conventional PTT. In recent years, numerous nanoparticles for cancer PTT have been investigated including gold nanostructures [6–22], carbon-based nanoparticles [23–40], magnetic nanoparticles [41–44], polymer nanospheres [45–47], polymer-coated chlorophyll nanoparticles [48], and semiconductor QDs [49–59], etc.

In this chapter, only the use of QDs in cancer PTT is discussed. QDs are fluorescent nanomaterials that have many advantages over traditional fluorescent dyes. Although QDs have been used in biomedical research for more than 18 years, most of the work has focused on fluorescence imaging. QDs exhibit a broad continuous excitation spectrum spanning from ultraviolet to NIR wavelength. Upon red or NIR laser irradiation, QDs that are brown or close to black in color not only generate reactive oxygen species (ROS), but also efficiently convert laser light into heat. The latter property can be used for cancer PTT.

2. Copper-based QDs for Photothermal Cancer Therapy

2.1 CuS nanocrystals

In 2003, Hirsch *et al.* [6] first used gold nanoshells for cancer PTT. From then on, numerous gold nanoparticles with various structures and other nanoparticles as mentioned above have been widely investigated for cancer PTT. However, gold nanostructures are usually relatively large. For example, NIR-absorbing gold nanoshells with a core diameter of 110 ± 11 nm and a 10 nm-thick gold shell have been reported [6]. The optimum diameter of nanoparticles for intravenous injection is between 10 and 50 nm [57, 60–62]. In addition, gold nanostructures are fabricated from an expensive noble metal, which may be undesirable for clinical applications.

Copper-based semiconductor nanoparticles are less expensive than gold nanoparticles, and exhibit low toxicity in biomedical detection and *in vivo* imaging [63–66]. Importantly, copper-based QDs have high optical absorption coefficients in the NIR region. In addition, some copper-based QDs are only several nanometers in diameter.

In 2010, Li *et al.* [59] found that the temperature of semiconductor CuS nanocrystals rapidly increased upon 808 nm laser irradiation, and could efficiently induce the destruction of human cervix adenocarcinoma HeLa cells. This was the first report on the use of copper-based QDs for cancer PTT. Li and co-workers synthesized thioglycolic acid (TGA)-stabilized CuS nanocrystals with an average diameter of approximately 3 nm composed of high-quality covellite CuS with hexagonal structure. The maximum absorption of the TGA-CuS was located at 900 nm, and the absorption coefficient at this wavelength was about $2 \times 10^7\ M^{-1}\ cm^{-1}$. The NIR absorption of the CuS nanocrystals was derived from *d–d* transitions of Cu^{2+} ions, which differ from the localized surface plasmon resonance (LSPR) displayed by gold nanostructures. The LSPR absorption of gold nanoparticles shifts when they migrate into cells because the dielectric constant of the surrounding medium has changed. In contrast, the *d–d* transition peaks of CuS nanocrystals located in the NIR band (900 nm) is not affected by the size and shape of the nanoparticles or the medium

[59, 67]. The absorption of CuS in the NIR band is advantageous because these nanocrystals can convert NIR laser light energy into heat. When 100 μL of an aqueous solution of TGA-CuS (770 μmol/L CuS QDs) was irradiated by a 808 nm laser (24 W/cm^2) for 5 min, the solution temperature increased by 12.7°C, whereas no obvious change in temperature of pure water was detected under the same irradiation conditions. When cancer cells were treated with the TGA-CuS QDs and laser irradiation, the extent of cell death strongly depended on the concentration of TGA-CuS QDs and the output power of the laser light. For example, after HeLa cells were incubated with 384 μmol/L of TGA-CuS QDs and irradiated at 808 nm (24 W/cm^2) for 5 min, the cell viability decreased from about 100% to 55.6 ± 5.8%. When the power density of the laser was increased up to 40 or 64 W/cm^2, the cell viability decreased to ~20% and ~15% after irradiation, respectively. In addition, these CuS nanocrystals exhibit low toxicity. When human embryonic kidney 293 cells were incubated with TGA-CuS QDs at concentrations of up to 100 μmol/L for 48 h, the cell viability did not obviously decrease.

However, the photothermal conversion efficiency of the TGA-stabilized CuS QDs described above is not high. To meet the demands of *in vivo* cancer PTT, copper-based nanocrystals with higher photothermal conversion efficiency need to be developed. In 2011, Tian *et al.* [58] synthesized copper chalcogenide nanocrystals composed of rhombohedral plate-like Cu_9S_5 with an average diameter of 70 nm and average thickness of ~13 nm (Fig. 6.1a). The Cu_9S_5 nanocrystal surfaces were capped with 6-aminocaproic acid (6-ACA). The 6-ACA-modified Cu_9S_5 nanocrystals were hydrophilic and displayed high stability in water (Fig. 6.1b, inset). The ACA-Cu_9S_5 nanocrystals strongly absorbed in the NIR region with high extinction coefficients (e.g., 1.2 × 10^9 M^{-1} cm^{-1} at 980 nm), as illustrated in Fig. 6.1b. Because Cu_9S_5 is a p-type semiconductor with a relatively high carrier (hole) concentration and strong free carrier absorption, the NIR absorbance of the Cu_9S_5 nanocrystals was mainly attributed to LSPR. When a series of aqueous solutions of the ACA-Cu_9S_5 nanocrystals (300 μL) with Cu^{2+} concentrations ranging from 1.2 to 40 ppm were irradiated at 980 nm (0.51 W/cm^2) for 7 min, the temperature of the solutions increased by 6.8–15.1°C from the initial

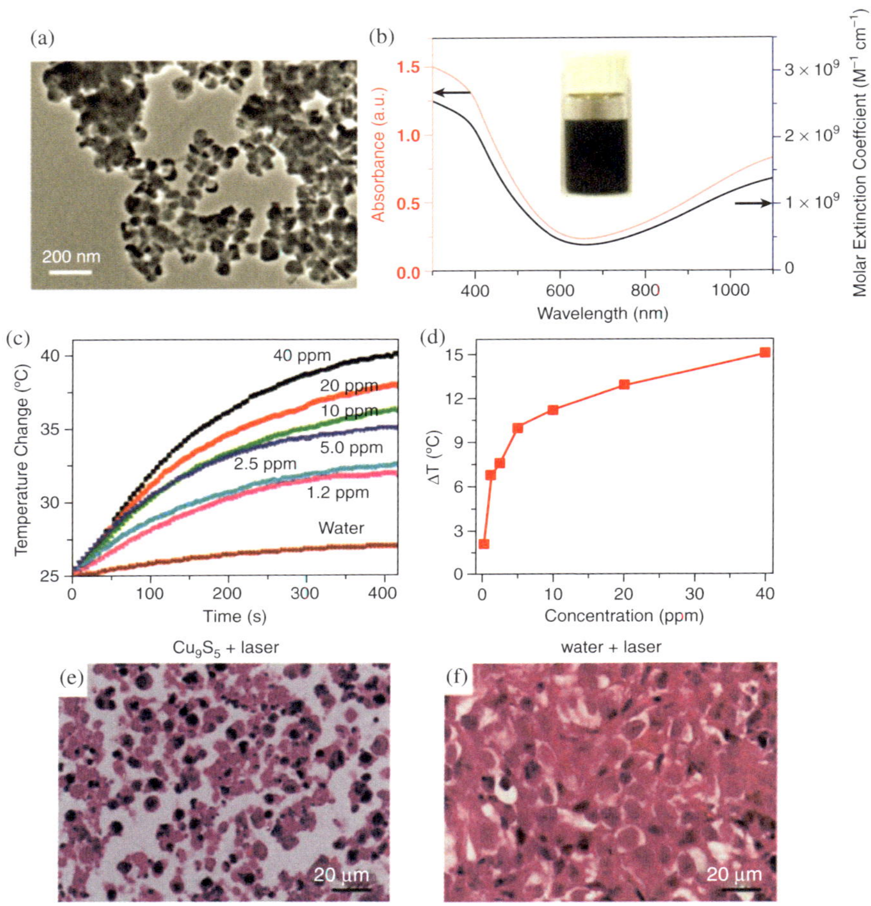

Fig. 6.1. (a) Transmission electron microscopy (TEM) image of 6-ACA-capped Cu_9S_5 nanocrystals. (b) Absorption spectrum (red line) and molar extinction coefficient (blue line) of an aqueous dispersion of hydrophilic Cu_9S_5 nanocrystals (40 ppm Cu^{2+}). The inset photograph shows the hydrophilic Cu_9S_5 nanocrystals in water after one week. (c) Temperature increase of Cu_9S_5 solutions (300 μL) with different concentrations of Cu^{2+} and pure water (control) upon 980 nm laser irradiation (0.51 W/cm^2). (d) Relationship between the temperature change (ΔT) over a period of 7 min and concentration (Cu^{2+}) of Cu_9S_5. Images of hematoxylin and eosin (H&E)-stained tumor tissue from mouse tumors injected with (e) 40 ppm of hydrophilic Cu_9S_5 and (f) water and then irradiated at 980 nm for 10 min. Reprinted with permission from Ref. [58]. Copyright (2011) American Chemical Society.

temperature of 25°C (Fig. 6.1c); the higher the concentration of Cu_9S_5 nanocrystals, the more rapid the temperature increase upon laser irradiation (Fig. 6.1d). The photothermal conversion efficiency of the ACA-Cu_9S_5 nanocrystals irradiated by the 980 nm laser was 25.7%. The temperature increase of the solutions containing the Cu_9S_5 nanocrystals was caused by their photothermal conversion because the temperature of pure water increased by less than 2.2°C under the same irradiation conditions (Fig. 6.1c). Because these Cu_9S_5 nanocrystals can rapidly and efficiently convert NIR laser light into heat energy, they may have the ability to kill cancer cells in living animals.

Tian and colleagues then injected 100 μL of the ACA-Cu_9S_5 nanocrystals (40 ppm) into tumors grown from human prostate carcinoma PC3 cells in mice and irradiated the tumors with a 980 nm laser at 0.51 W/cm^2 for 10 min [58]. They found that the tumor tissues were seriously damaged by this treatment, observing changes such as shrinking of malignant cells, loss of contact and nuclear damage (Fig. 6.1e). This was in stark contrast to the control experiment where tumors were treated with water and laser irradiation, which did not change the size or shape of the cancer cells in the tumor tissue (Fig. 6.1f). In addition, when the ACA-Cu_9S_5 nanocrystals with concentrations ranging from 1.6 to 50 ppm were incubated with human cervical carcinoma Hela cells for 24 h without laser irradiation, the cell viability did not obviously decrease. Overall, these ACA-Cu_9S_5 nanocrystals with high photothermal conversion efficiency and low cytotoxicity have considerable advantages for cancer PTT over the TGA-capped CuS nanocrystals described above.

The photothermal conversion efficiency of nanocrystals can be further enhanced by changing the stabilizer on the nanocrystal surfaces and/or the composition of the nanocrystals. In 2014, Liu *et al.* [50] used L-cysteine (Cys) as a stabilizer to synthesize CuS nanocrystals. Cys is an amino acid found in human beings, and is much safer than TGA and ACA. The photothermal conversion efficiency of the Cys–CuS nanocrystals reached 38.0% when they were irradiated with a 980 nm laser, which was much higher than that of the ACA-Cu_9S_5 nanocrystals (25.7%) described above. The as-prepared Cys–CuS nanocrystals were close to spherical with a diameter of ~18 nm. These nanocrystals may aggregate into small clusters in water because their average hydrodynamic diameter measured by dynamic light scattering was ~152.9 nm. The CuS nanocrystals were standard CuS phase with hexagonal structure, which was confirmed by X-ray diffraction measurements. The Fourier transform infrared spectrum of the Cys–CuS nanocrystals confirmed that Cys molecules were successfully used to cap the CuS surfaces. The Cys–CuS nanocrystals exhibited strong absorption in the NIR region with an absorption maxima at 1010 nm. When aqueous solutions of the Cys–CuS nanocrystals (300 μL) with Cu^{2+} concentrations of 5, 10, 25, 50, and 100 ppm were irradiated with a 980 nm laser (0.72 W/cm^2), the temperatures of the solutions increased by 8.4 to 21.5°C after 300 s. Meanwhile, the temperature of a control solution of 300 μL of pure water increased only by 3.8°C under the same irradiation conditions. To investigate the photothermal conversion of the Cys–CuS nanocrystals in animal tumors, mice with osteosarcoma grown from K7M2 cells were intratumorally injected with 0.10 mL of Cys–CuS nanocrystals (50 ppm Cu^{2+}) and then irradiated at 980 nm. After 300 s of irradiation, the surface temperature of the mouse tumor rapidly increased by about 20°C from the initial temperature of 31.8°C, which was a larger increase than that of the control group [tumor + phosphate-buffered saline (PBS) + laser]. These results indicate that the Cys–CuS nanocrystals may be useful for *in vivo* deep tumor treatment. When osteosarcoma-bearing mice were intratumorally injected with 150 μL of Cys–CuS solutions (50 ppm Cu^{2+}) and then irradiated at 980 nm for 10 min each day, tumor growth was greatly inhibited compared with that of the control group (tumor + PBS + laser) after 12 days of irradiation. This suggests that upon NIR laser irradiation, the Cys–CuS nanocrystals can readily kill *in vivo* cancer cells through photothermal conversion.

To further improve the photothermal conversion efficiency of copper-based nanocrystals, Li *et al.* [51] synthesized another kind of CuS with different components from the nanocrystals described above. These copper-based nanocrystals had the formula $Cu_{7.2}S_4$ and a mean size of ~20 nm. To obtain water-soluble nanocrystals, the $Cu_{7.2}S_4$ surfaces were coated with an amphiphilic hydrolyzed polymaleic anhydride premodified with oleylamine. The resulting polymer-coated $Cu_{7.2}S_4$ nanocrystals displayed an absorption maxima at 968 nm in wavelength. In addition, these hydrophilic nanocrystals may exhibit good monodispersity because their absorption intensity at 980 nm increased linearly as the concentration of $Cu_{7.2}S_4$ nanocrystals in water was increased. Importantly, these polymer-coated $Cu_{7.2}S_4$ nanocrystals readily converted 980 nm laser light (0.72 W/cm^2) into heat. The photothermal conversion efficiency of the polymer-coated $Cu_{7.2}S_4$ nanocrystals upon 980 nm laser irradiation was 56.7%. This suggests that cancer cells should be destroyed by a low dosage of the $Cu_{7.2}S_4$ nanocrystals upon NIR laser irradiation. Therefore, these polymer-coated $Cu_{7.2}S_4$ nanocrystals may be an excellent photothermal agent for cancer therapy.

Further experiments revealed that the polymer-coated $Cu_{7.2}S_4$ nanocrystals could also strongly convert NIR laser light into heat energy inside animal tumors. For example, when 100 μL of the polymer-coated $Cu_{7.2}S_4$ nanocrystals (40 ppm Cu^{2+}) were intratumorally injected into a mouse with an osteosarcoma grown from K7M2 cells and irradiated with the 980 nm laser, the temperature of the tumor surface increased rapidly to 43.4°C after 30 s and 46.0°C after 60 s. Severe cellular damage was observed in the treated tumor tissue. In contrast, the tumor temperature did not increase much and no cancer cell damage was detected for the control mouse with a tumor that was injected with PBS and then irradiated under the same conditions.

Constructing a superstructure of CuS crystals may improve their NIR absorption. Several years ago, an interesting flower-like CuS superstructure with high photothermal conversion efficiency in the NIR band was developed by Tian's group [56]. They prepared dark-green three-dimensional flower-like CuS superstructures with a diameter of ~1.5–3 μm by heated copper(II) chloride, sodium sulfide and poly(vinylpyrrolidone) at 180°C for 48 h. Careful observation revealed that these flowers were composed of intersectional hexagonal nanoplates with a mean edge length and thickness of ~500–800 nm and ~50 nm, respectively. The CuS flowers strongly absorbed in the NIR region, with an absorption intensity that was about twice that of their component CuS hexagonal nanoplates. After being irradiated with a NIR laser (e.g., 980 nm laser), the CuS flowers can serve as laser-cavity mirrors. This may be the reason why the CuS superstructures exhibit strong NIR absorption. The temperature of the CuS flowers increased more rapidly than that of the CuS hexagonal nanoplates when they were irradiated at 980 nm (0.51 W/cm^2), and the photothermal conversion efficiency of the CuS flowers was about 50%. *In vitro* and *in vivo* experiments showed that the CuS flowers could be used for cancer PTT. To investigate the ability of the NIR laser to penetrate tissue and the CuS flowers to kill cancer cells *in vitro* upon laser irradiation, HeLa cells were incubated with 2.5 g/L of the CuS flowers and the cells were then covered with chicken skin (thickness: ~1 mm). After being irradiated with the 980 nm laser for 5 min, most of the cancer cells were dead, whereas laser irradiation alone did not obviously affect cell viability. Animal experiments using mouse with tumors grown from PC-3 human prostate cancer cells showed that treatment with the CuS flowers and 980 nm laser irradiation caused marked degenerative changes and coagulative necrosis. However, these CuS flowers are too large for targeted delivery *in vivo*, which may prevent their use in targeted cancer PTT.

If CuS nanocrystals are loaded with drugs, the resulting nanocomposites obtained may be used as multifunctional materials for multimodal therapy or imaging. In 2013, Song *et al.* [52] coated Cu_9S_5 nanocrystals with mesoporous silica ($mSiO_2$) shells and PEG layers to stabilize the nanoparticles and enhance their blood compatibility. The $mSiO_2$ shells can not only reduce the toxicity of the CuS cores and improve the hydrophilicity of CuS, but also render the nanocrystals drug carriers. The pore volume of the obtained Cu_9S_5@$mSiO_2$-PEG core–shell nanostructures (~45 nm in diameter) was very high (0.224 cm^3/g). This allowed anticancer drug doxorubicin (DOX) to be incorporated into the Cu_9S_5@$mSiO_2$-PEG nanocomposites. The encapsulation efficiency and loading content of DOX within the nanocomposites were 63.8% and 13.76%, respectively. These DOX-loaded Cu_9S_5@$mSiO_2$-PEG nanocomposites may be synchronously used for cancer chemotherapy and PTT. For example, when Hep3B hepatocarcinoma cells were incubated with the nanocomposites and free DOX and then irradiated with a 980 nm laser (0.72 W/cm^2), the cell viability in the experiments with DOX-loaded Cu_9S_5@$mSiO_2$-PEG and laser irradiation was much lower than that in experiments with equivalent concentrations of free DOX and DOX-loaded Cu_9S_5@mSiO_2-PEG without irradiation and Cu_9S_5@mSiO_2-PEG with laser exposure. The synergistic effect of the chemotherapy and PTT of the DOX-loaded Cu_9S_5@mSiO_2-PEG nanocomposites was also demonstrated in animal experiments. Mouse tumors grown from human colon carcinoma cells HCT 116 were injected with DOX-loaded Cu_9S_5@mSiO_2-PEG and then irradiated with the laser. This markedly inhibited tumor growth compared with that in the control group. Drug-loaded CuS nanocrystals can not only be used for multimodal cancer therapies, but also for *in vivo* cancer imaging. This is because CuS may act as an infrared thermal imaging agent, and is also suitable for photoacoustic imaging.

2.2 CuSe and CuTe nanocrystals

CuSe and CuTe can also generate sufficient photothermal heating for cancer PTT by NIR laser irradiation. In 2011, Hessel *et al.* [57] synthesized $Cu_{2-x}Se$ nanocrystals as a photothermal agent by arrested precipitation in a hot organic solvent (Fig. 6.2a). The as-prepared $Cu_{2-x}Se$ nanocrystals were spherical, with an average diameter of 16 ± 1 nm (Fig. 6.2b). To obtain water-soluble nanocrystals, the surfaces of the $Cu_{2-x}Se$ particles were coated with an amphiphilic polymer composed of a poly(maleic anhydride) backbone with hydrophilic carboxylic acid groups and hydrophobic oleylamine side chains. The resulting polymer-coated $Cu_{2-x}Se$ nanocrystals had an average hydrodynamic diameter of 39 nm. These polymer-coated $Cu_{2-x}Se$ nanocrystals exhibited broad strong absorption in the NIR band with a maxima at 970 nm (Fig. 6.2c). The molar extinction coefficient of the $Cu_{2-x}Se$ nanocrystals reached 7.7×10^7 M^{-1} cm^{-1} at 970 nm. The photothermal conversion efficiency of the $Cu_{2-x}Se$ nanocrystals irradiated by an 800 nm laser was 22%, which was higher than that of commercial Au nanoshells (13%) and nanorods (21%). Cell experiments revealed that most human colorectal cancer cells (HCT-116) died after they were treated with the polymer-coated $Cu_{2-x}Se$ nanocrystals and then irradiated at 800 nm laser (30 W/cm^2) for 5 min.

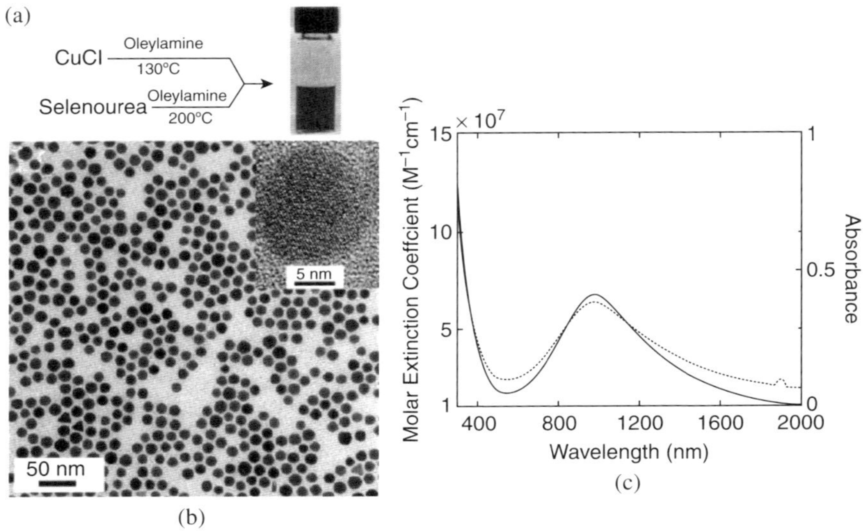

Fig. 6.2. (a) Formation of oleylamine-capped $Cu_{2-x}Se$ nanocrystals in a hot organic solvent and a photograph of a dispersion of the nanocrystals in chloroform. (b) TEM image of the $Cu_{2-x}Se$ nanocrystals. (c) Absorption (dotted line) and molar extinction coefficient (solid line) of the polymer-coated $Cu_{2-x}Se$ nanocrystals. Reprinted with permission from Ref. [57]. Copyright (2011) American Chemical Society.

In 2013, Li *et al.* [54] developed CuTe nanocrystals with NIR absorption and different morphologies for cancer PTT. CuTe nanocubes, nanoplates and nanorods, as shown in Figs. 6.3a–6.3c, respectively, were obtained by controlling the nominal ratio of Cu to Te, the reaction time and temperature, and the concentration of trioctylphosphine stabilizer. These nanocrystals have narrow size distributions. All of the CuTe nanocrystals exhibited an absorption band centered at 900 nm, but the intensity of this band for the CdTe nanocubes was weaker than that for the nanoplates and nanorods (Fig. 6.3d), which indicated that the NIR absorption of the CuTe nanocrystals was controlled by their geometry. Upon NIR laser irradiation, these polymer-coated CuTe nanocrystals could efficiently kill 3T3 embryonic fibroblast cells.

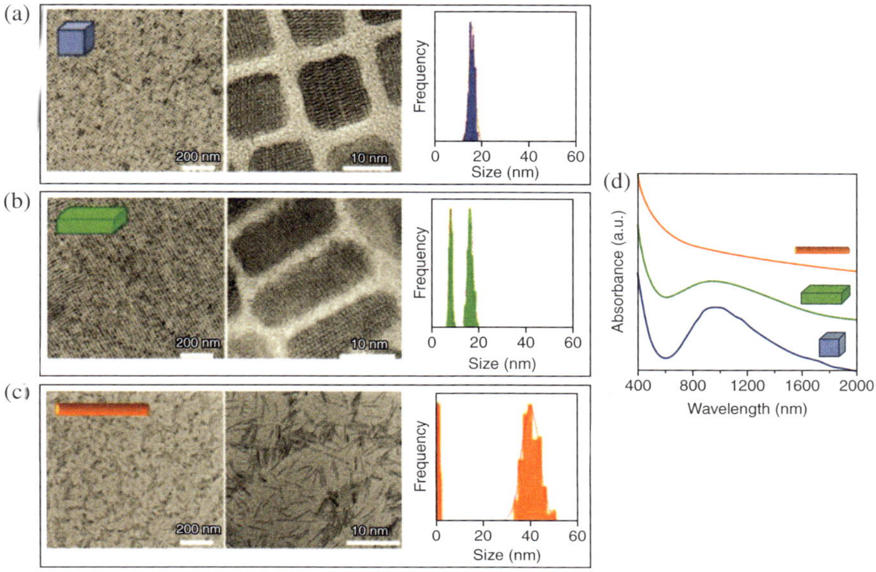

Fig. 6.3. (a–c) TEM images (left: low magnification, right: high magnification) and size distributions of CuTe (a) nanocubes, (b) nanoplates and (c) nanorods. (d) Absorption spectra of the CuTe nanocubes, nanoplates and nanorods. Reprinted with permission from Ref. [54]. Copyright (2013) American Chemical Society.

3. Cadmium Selenide and Cadmium Telluride QDs for Photothermal Cancer Therapy

3.1 Reducing the toxicity of cadmium-containing QDs by coating with a silica shell

Besides copper-based QDs, the commonly used cadmium (Cd)-containing QDs such as cadmium selenide (CdSe) and cadmium telluride (CdTe) that emit red or NIR fluorescence also have potential for cancer PTT. Cd-containing QDs are toxic to cells and animals because they release cadmium ions (Cd^{2+}), which are potentially hazardous because of their neurological, renal and liver toxicity, and have even been found to be carcinogenic. Therefore, researchers have tried to limit the release of

Cd ions from QDs by modifying the QDs via numerous techniques. Typically, a shell is fabricated on the QD surface, which may be a polymer, liposome, or rigid inorganic layer. Many reports have shown that silicon nanoparticles are nontoxic and biodegradable *in vivo* [68–70]. A silica (SiO_2) shell is biocompatible, optically transparent, and easy to form on QDs. QDs coated with SiO_2 exhibit low toxicity compared with uncoated QDs [55, 71] and those coated with organic matrix (e.g., liposomes). Silica-coated QDs can be synthesized in a quaternary water-in-oil microemulsion system [72]. The thickness and density of the three-dimensional network of the SiO_2 shell could be controlled by varying the reaction rate and the amount of tetraethyl orthosilicate (TEOS) in the precursor. Figure 6.4 shows a TEM image of a CdSe/SiO_2 sample synthesized in the microemulsion system. QDs are located in the centre of the nanospheres to form a core–shell structure. When 3 mL of this CdSe/SiO_2 sample (containing about 54.54 μmol Cd^{2+} ions) was dialyzed against 40 mL of an aqueous solution (0.9% NaCl) as a receptor phase at pH 8.50 for 1 week, the

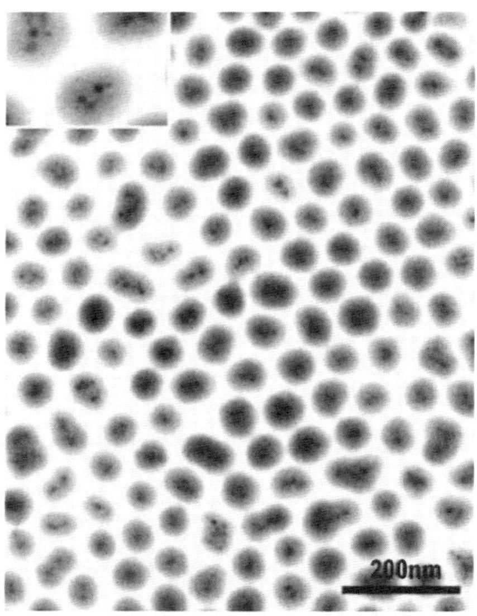

Fig. 6.4. TEM image of the CdSe/SiO_2 QDs synthesized in a quaternary water-in-oil microemulsion system. The inset shows an enlarged view. Reprinted with permission from Ref. [72]. Copyright (2007) Springer.

concentration of accumulated Cd^{2+} ions in the receptor phase was only 0.84 ppm. When the pH of the receptor phase was decreased to 7.3, the release rate of Cd^{2+} ions decreased (no more than 0.25 ppm after 1 week of dialysis) compared with the case at higher pH. When strong acid solution with a pH of 2.02 was used as the receptor phase, the concentration of Cd^{2+} ions in the receptor phase was no more than 0.5 ppm after 1 week of dialysis. In contrast, when the uncoated CdSe were dialyzed against physiological saline, the concentration of Cd^{2+} ions released from the QDs increased rapidly with dialysis time. For example, when CdSe QDs with same concentration as CdSe/SiO_2 above were dialyzed for 1 week, the concentrations of Cd^{2+} ions in the receptor phases at pH of 8.50, 7.30 and 2.02 were 5.25, 8.42, and 121.35 ppm, respectively. These values indicate that many more Cd^{2+} ions were released from the uncoated CdSe QDs than from the CdSe/SiO_2 QDs under the same conditions. In addition, coating the QD surfaces with thicker SiO_2 shells would further inhibit the release of toxic Cd^{2+}.

It should be noted that no shells completely prevented the QDs from releasing toxic ions. A small amount of Cd^{2+} ions in the receptor solution could be detected when the CdSe/SiO_2 were dialyzed against physiological saline, which implied that the SiO_2 shells of the CdSe/SiO_2 spheres contained pores. The CdSe/SiO_2 shown in Fig. 6.4 contain micropores with diameters ranging from 0.58 to 0.91 nm (Fig. 6.5), and their specific surface

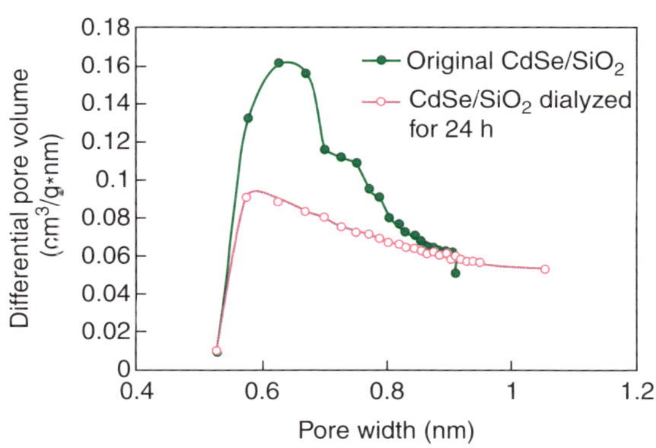

Fig. 6.5. Pore sizes distributions of CdSe/SiO_2 before and after dialysis against an aqueous solution at pH 7.30 containing 0.9% NaCl for 24 h. Reprinted with permission from Ref. [72]. Copyright (2007) Springer.

area was more than 200 m^2/g, as determined by the Horvath–Kawazoe and Brunauer–Emmett–Teller methods. These pores allow Cd^{2+} ions to escape from the CdSe/SiO_2 QDs. However, the release rate of Cd^{2+} ions from the CdSe/SiO_2 QDs in a solution at pH 7.3 gradually leveled off over the next week of dialysis. This is because the micropore volume of the CdSe/SiO_2 decreased after dialysis (Fig. 6.5), so the relatively small micropores may be blocked by the Cd^{2+} ions released from the CdSe cores. Despite some limitations of the SiO_2 matrix, using a SiO_2 shell to coating the surface of QDs may still be a good strategy to reduce QD toxicity.

SiO_2-coated QDs should be well dispersed in aqueous solution and remain soluble in the water phase for a long time for use as bioimaging probes and therapy reagents. The SiO_2-coated QDs with an appropriate thickness of silica shell formed from the reaction between water-soluble QDs and TEOS in aqueous solution are usually stable in water. For example, when the TEOS solutions (containing 20% [v/v] of ethanol) were directly added into aqueous solutions of mercaptopropionic acid (MPA)-capped CdTe QDs with an emission maxima of 710 nm to synthesize CdTe/SiO_2 nanocomposites the resulting CdTe(710)/SiO_2 core–shell nanospheres dispersed well in aqueous solution [55]. The formation of SiO_2 shells was confirmed by TEM, energy-dispersive X-ray spectroscopy and the difference in the diameters of CdTe(710) and CdTe(710)/SiO_2, respectively. The release rate of Cd from the SiO_2-coated CdTe(710) was effectively delayed by coating with a thicker SiO_2 shell. When the CdTe(710) were dialyzed against PBS for 5 h, about $1.47 \pm 0.10\%$ of the Cd was lost from the uncoated QDs, whereas only about $0.94 \pm 0.04\%$, $0.47 \pm 0.01\%$, and $0.36 \pm 0.01\%$ of Cd was released from the CdTe(710)/SiO_2 with SiO_2 shells with thicknesses of 0.48 ± 0.32, 2.19 ± 1.10 and 3.45 ± 1.51 nm, respectively. This indicates that coating QDs with a SiO_2 shell helps to protect them from degradation. As a result, the toxicity of the QDs to the surrounding environment may be decreased by the SiO_2 shell minimizing the release of Cd from the QD cores.

Cell experiments demonstrated that the CdTe(710)/SiO_2 QDs exhibited lower toxicity to both normal and cancer cells than the uncoated CdTe(710) QDs. For example, when normal liver cells (QSG-7701) and melanoma cells (A375) were incubated with CdTe(710)/SiO_2 QDs (0.05 mg/mL) for 12 h, the cell viabilities were $86.75 \pm 8.99\%$ and $80.98 \pm$

19.93%, respectively. Conversely, when the normal liver and melanoma cells were incubated with the uncoated CdTe(710) QDs for 12 h, the viabilities of both normal and cancer cells obviously decreased and were significantly lower ($p < 0.05$) than those of the cells incubated with CdTe(710)/SiO_2 QDs. The toxic effects of CdTe(710)/SiO_2 on *in vitro* cultured normal and cancer cells were more pronounced than those on cells in living animals. This is because the environmental conditions for *in vitro* cell growth in culture were harsher than those in living animals.

3.2 Photothermal conversion of cadmium-containing QDs upon NIR laser irradiation

The photothermal conversion efficiency of nanomaterials is related to the absorption coefficient of the nanomaterials at the wavelength of the laser light. The higher the absorption coefficient, the higher the photothermal conversion efficiency. However, the absorption spectra of Cd-containing QDs do not usually extend to longer than 750 nm. The absorption coefficient of Cd-containing QDs at wavelengths >700 nm is low. A laser with a wavelength no more than 700 nm is therefore suitable for inducing the photothermal conversion of such QDs. Although the ability of photons of laser light with a wavelength of ≤ 700 nm to propagate through living tissue is low compared with those of laser light that is ≥ 700 nm, many clinical and animal experiments have demonstrated that laser light ranging from 650 to 700 nm can be successfully used for cancer phototherapy [55, 73–75].

Fig. 6.6 shows aqueous solutions of six different CdTe QDs and their temperature increase upon laser irradiation. The emission maxima of these CdTe were 534, 561, 596, 626, 660 to 710 nm, so their fluorescence changed gradually from green to deep red (Fig. 6.6a). The temperatures of all the QD solutions gradually increased over time during 671 nm laser irradiation. The temperature increases induced by the more deeply colored QDs (those with longer emission maxima) were larger than those caused by the lighter colored QDs (those with shorter emission maxima). For example, when the CdTe QDs (200 μL, 2 mg/mL) with emission maxima of 534, 561, 596, 626, 660 to 710 nm were irradiated by a 671 nm laser (power density: 0.2 W/cm^2), the average temperature of the QD solutions

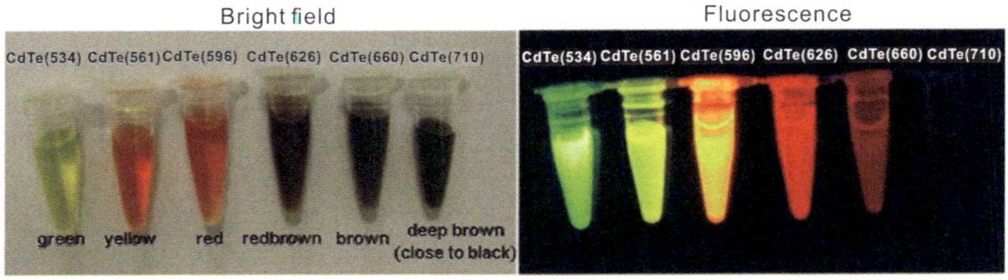

(a)

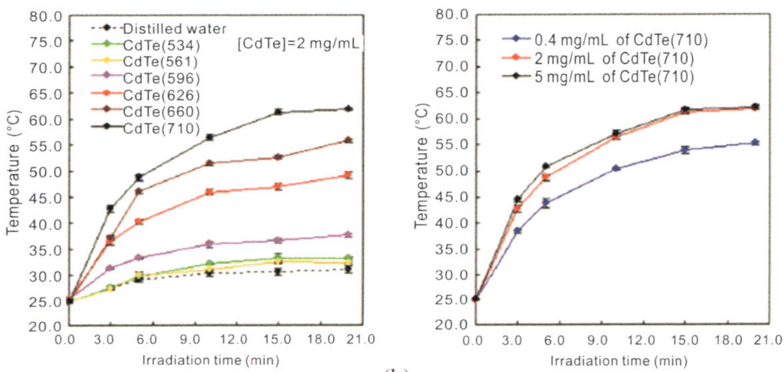

(b)

Fig. 6.6. (a) Bright-field and corresponding fluorescence images of aqueous solutions of CdTe QDs with different emission maxima. (b) Temperature increases of aqueous solutions of (left) CdTe with different emission maxima (2 mg/mL) and (right) different concentrations of CdTe with an emission maxima of 710 nm upon 671 nm laser irradiation. Reprinted with permission from Ref. [55]. Copyright (2012) Elsevier.

increased rapidly during the initial 5 min, and increased by over 8.5, 7.5, 12.4, 23.9, 31.1, and 36.9°C, respectively, from the initial temperature of 25°C after 20 min of irradiation (Fig. 6.6b, left). In addition, the temperature of the CdTe QD solutions with higher concentration increased more rapidly during laser irradiation than that of QD solutions with low concentration (Fig. 6.6b, right). Meanwhile, the average temperature of 200 μL of distilled water only increased about 6.1°C after 20 min of irradiation (Fig. 6.6b, left). These results show that CdTe QDs can convert 671 nm laser light into heat. Furthermore, after coating with a SiO_2 shell, the resulting CdTe/SiO_2 could also efficiently convert laser light into heat, and the SiO_2 shells had only a minor effect on the temperature increase. For example, the temperatures of solutions of CdTe(710)/SiO_2 with SiO_2 shells of different thicknesses (0.48–3.45 nm) were only 1.7–2.6°C lower than that of the uncoated CdTe(710) after 20 min of 671 nm laser irradiation.

CdSe QDs can also efficiently convert laser light into heat energy. For example, when a solution of CdSe (200 μL, 2 mg/mL) with an emission maxima of 609 nm was irradiated at 671 nm for 20 min, the average temperature of the solution increased by over 22.3°C from the initial 25°C. However, the absorption onsets of CdSe are usually located at short wavelength. Therefore, improving the photothermal conversion efficiency of CdSe in the NIR region is more difficult than for CdTe.

Upon laser irradiation, QDs can not only generate heat, but also produce ROS. As shown in Fig. 6.7, both SiO_2-coated and uncoated CdTe QDs with an emission maxima at 710 nm could effectively generate intracellular ROS when the QDs were incubated with human melanoma cells (A375) and irradiated with a 671 nm laser. The level of ROS increased with both QD concentration and laser irradiation time during the initial 20 min. It is known that ROS tend to induce cell destruction and death through the photooxidation of DNA and proteins in cells. This is the basic principle of photodynamic therapy (PDT). Therefore, QDs can act as photothermal reagents for cancer PTT, as well as photosensitizers for cancer PDT. QDs with PDT capability would exhibit increased effectiveness for PTT. Other photothermal reagents such as gold nanostructures are usually combined with photosensitizers to obtain an additive or synergistic effect during cancer therapy. However, NIR QDs do not need to conjugate with additional photosensitizer because these semiconductor nanocrystals synchronously possess the capabilities of PTT and PDT.

Because the CdTe(710)/SiO_2 QDs introduced above displayed high photothermal conversion efficiency, the use of these QDs in cancer phototherapy was investigated [55]. The growth of the tumors (length and width before first irradiation: 4–5 mm) grew from A375 melanoma cells was strongly inhibited when the tumors were injected with the CdTe(710)/SiO_2 (50 μL, 5 mg/mL) and irradiated with a 671 nm laser for 20 min every 24 h, and all the mouse tumors ($n = 5$) had disappeared 18 days from the start of irradiation. Furthermore, there was no tumor recurrence at the

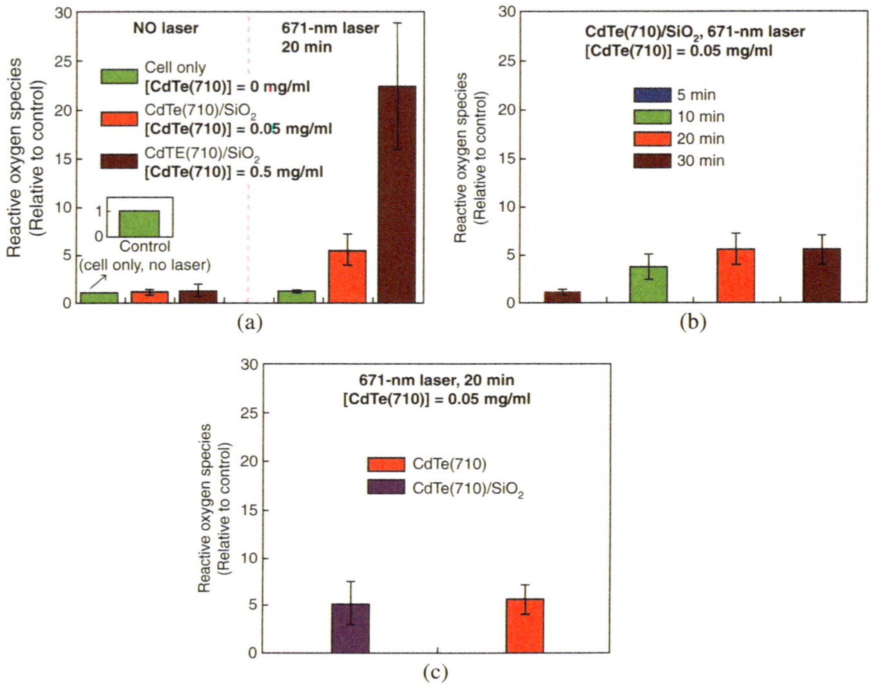

Fig. 6.7. Influence of (a) CdTe(671) concentration, (b) irradiation time and (c) a SiO_2 shell on the intracellular level of ROS in A375 human melanoma cells generated by CdTe(710) with and without a SiO_2 shell upon 671 nm laser irradiation. Reprinted with permission from Ref. [55]. Copyright (2012) Elsevier.

original tumor sites after the termination of laser irradiation. This indicated that the cancer cells were completely killed at the tumor sites by treatment with the CdTe(710)/SiO_2 and laser irradiation. Investigation of the pathological changes in tumor tissues caused by treatment with CdTe(710)/SiO_2 and laser irradiation showed that the cancer cells and tumor blood vessels were severely damaged following irradiation for three days (20 min daily). Meanwhile, the tumors of mice in control groups grew normally over this time, and no obvious damage was detected on the skin of the tumor. The inhibition of tumor growth caused by the CdTe(710)/SiO_2 QDs and laser irradiation may be the synergistic effect of PTT and PDT of the QDs.

4. Discussion

Semiconductor QDs are only several nanometers in diameter. Such small nanoparticles usually possess high surface energy, which allows them to bind strongly to cancer cell surfaces. The cell membrane can be damaged by the heat generated by the QDs when they are irradiated with red or NIR light. The damaged cell membrane can then release cell contents such as intracellular calcium ions. Small-sized QDs can also easily penetrate into cancer cells. In general, most nanoparticles first migrate into lysosomes and then remain in this organelle for a long time. Lysosomes are acidic organelles (pH ~5) that contain a large amount of digestive enzymes. Once lysosomes are damaged by the photothermal effect of QDs, the release of lysosomal contents will cause cell death because the released enzymes and lowered cytoplasmic pH will destroy DNA and protein structures. In addition, QDs can also produce ROS and release toxic metal ions upon laser irradiation, which help to improve the efficacy of cancer PTT.

Semiconductor quantum rods (QRs) can also convert NIR light into heat because QRs with suitable width and length strongly absorb in the NIR band. Aqueous solutions of these NIR QRs are usually deep red, brown, or close to black in color. Upon exposure to NIR laser irradiation, NIR QRs may also generate ROS. The efficacy of phototherapy using QRs may be similar to that using QDs. Although little work has been reported on cancer phototherapy using QRs, an increasing number of researchers may investigate this possibility in the near future, because the optical properties of QRs are advantageous over those of QDs.

QDs and QRs upon NIR laser irradiation exhibit multimodal therapies, which can be illustrated in Fig. 6.8. Therefore, these multifunctional nanomaterials have been attracting great attention worldwide.

However, semiconductor QDs and QRs are both composed of heavy metals. Cd-containing QDs and QRs are toxic to both cancer and normal cells. Once such nonbiodegradable nanoparticles are taken up by a living cell, they are not easily released by it. The toxicity of QDs and QRs currently limits their *in vivo* applications. Therefore, developing low-toxicity QDs and QRs and improving their photothermal conversion efficiencies are necessary to promote the use of QDs and QRs in cancer PTT.

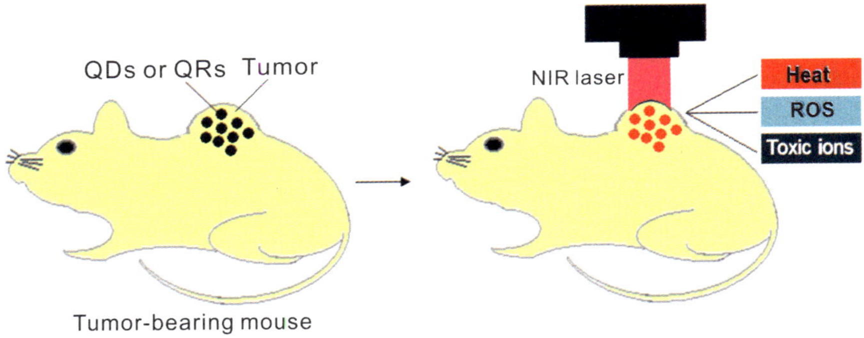

Fig. 6.8. Schematic illustration of the NIR laser triggered QDs or QRs for cancer multimodal therapies (PTT + PDT + toxicity of ions released from the QDs or QRs).

Decreasing the injection dosage of low-toxicity QDs/QRs with high photothermal conversion efficiency may be a good strategy to realize clinical cancer PTT using QDs/QRs.

References

[1] Reinhold HS and Endrich B. (1986). Tumour microcirculation as a target for hyperthermia. *Biomaterials*, **2**:111–137.

[2] Raaphorst, G. P. Fundamental aspects of hyperthermic biology. In Field SB, Hand JW. *An introduction to the practical aspects of clinical hyperthermia*, London. Taylor & Francis; 1990. pp. 10–54.

[3] Fajardo LF. (1984). Pathological effects of hyperthermia in normal tissues. *Cancer Res.*, **44**:4826–4835.

[4] van der Zee J. (2002). Heating the patient: a promising approach? *Ann. Oncol.*, **13**:1173–1184.

[5] Jaque D, Martinez Maestro L, del Rosal B, Haro-Gonzalez P, Benayas A, Plaza JL, Rodríguez EM and Solé JG. (2014). Nanoparticles for photothermal therapies. *Nanoscale*, **6**:9494–9530.

[6] Hirsch LR, Stafford RJ, Bankson JA, Sershen SR, Rivera B, Price RE, Hazle JD, Halas NJ and West JL. (2003). Nanoshell-mediated near-infrared thermal therapy of tumors under magnetic resonance guidance. *Proc. Natl. Acad. Sci. USA*, **100**:13549–13554.

[7] Jin H, Liu X, Gui R and Wang Z. (2015). Facile synthesis of gold nanorods/hydrogels core/shell nanospheres for pH and near-infrared-light induced release of 5-fluorouracil and chemo-photothermal therapy. *Colloids Surf B Biointerfaces*, **128**:498–505.

[8] Kannadorai RK, Chiew GGY, Luo KQ and Liu Q. (2015). Dual functions of gold nanorods as photothermal agent and autofluorescence enhancer to track cell death during plasmonicphotothermal therapy. *Cancer Lett.*, **357**:152–159.

[9] Ayala-Orozco C, Urban C, Bishnoi S, Urban A, Charron H, Mitchell T, Shea M, Nanda S, Schiff R, Halas N and Joshi A. (2014) Sub-100 nm gold nanomatryoshkas improve photo-thermal therapy efficacy in large and highly aggressive triple negative breast tumors. *J. Controlled Release*, **191**:90–97.

[10] Seo SH, Kim BM, Joe A, Han HW, Chen X, Cheng Z and Jang ES. (2014). NIR-light-induced surface-enhanced Raman scattering for detection and photothermal/photodynamic therapy of cancer cells using methylene blue-embedded gold nanorod@SiO2 nanocomposites. *Biomaterials*, **35**:3309–3318.

[11] Wang B, Wang JH, Liu Q, Huang H, Chen M, Li K, Li CZ, Yu XF and Chu PK. (2014). Rose-bengal-conjugated gold nanorods for *in vivo* photodynamic and photothermal oral cancer therapies. *Biomaterials*, **35**:1954–1966.

[12] Okuno T, Kato S, Hatakeyama Y, Okajima J, Maruyama S, Sakamoto M, Mori S and Kodama T. (2013). Photothermal therapy of tumors in lymph nodes using gold nanorods and near-infrared laser light. *J. Control Release*, **172**:879–884.

[13] Yang HW, Liu HL, Li ML, Hsi IW, Fan CT, Huang CY, Lu YJ, Hua MY, Chou HY, Liaw JW, Ma CC and Wei KC. (2013). Magnetic gold-nanorod/PNIPAAmMA nanoparticles for dual magnetic resonance and photoacoustic imaging and targeted photothermal therapy. *Biomaterials*, **34**:5651–5660.

[14] Jin Y, Wang J, Ke H, Wang S and Dai Z. (2013). Graphene oxide modified PLA microcapsules containing gold nanoparticles for ultrasonic/CT bimodal imaging guided photothermal tumor therapy. *Biomaterials*, **34**:4794–4802.

[15] Shen S, Tang H, Zhang X, Ren J, Pang Z, Wang D, Gao H, Qian Y, Jiang X and Yang W. (2013). Targeting mesoporous silica-encapsulated gold nanorods

for chemo-photothermal therapy with near-infrared radiation. *Biomaterials*, **34**:3150–3158.

[16] Wang Y, Black KC, Luehmann H, Li W, Zhang Y, Cai X, Wan D, Liu SY, Li M, Kim P, Li ZY, Wang LV, Liu Y and Xia Y. (2013). Comparison study of gold nanohexapods, nanorods, and nanocages for photothermal cancer treatment. *ACS Nano*, **7**:2068–2077.

[17] Yu C, Wo F, Shao Y, Dai X and Chu M. (2013). Bovine serum albumin nanospheres synchronously encapsulating gold selenium/gold nanoparticles and photosensitizer for high-efficiency cancer phototherapy. *Appl. Biochem. Biotechnol.*, **169**:1566–1578.

[18] Kuo WS, Chang YT, Cho KC, Chiu KC, Lien CH, Yeh CS and Chen SJ. (2012). Gold nanomaterials conjugated with indocyanine green for dual-modality photodynamic and photothermal therapy. *Biomaterials*, **33**:3270–3278.

[19] Chen J, Glaus C, Laforest R, Zhang Q, Yang M, Gidding M, Welch MJ and Xia Y. (2010). Gold nanocages as photothermal transducers for cancer treatment. *Small*, **6**:811–817.

[20] Dickerson EB, Dreaden EC, Huang X, El-Sayed IH, Chu H, Pushpanketh S, McDonald JF and El-Sayed MA. (2008). Gold nanorod assisted near-infrared plasmonic photothermal therapy (PPTT) of squamous cell carcinoma in mice. *Cancer Lett.*, **269**:57–66.

[21] Tanya S. Hauck, Jennings TL, Yatsenko T, Kumaradas JC and Chan WCW. (2008). Enhancing the toxicity of cancer chemotherapeutics with gold nanorod hyperthermia. *Adv. Mater.*, **20**:3832–3838.

[22] Chen J, Wang D, Xi J, Au L, Siekkinen A, Warsen A, Li ZY, Zhang H, Xia Y and Li X. (2007). Immuno gold nanocages with tailored optical properties for targeted photothermal destruction of cancer cells. *Nano Lett.*, **7**:1318–1322.

[23] Wang H, Sun Y, Yi J, Fu J, Di J, Del Carmen Alonso A and Zhou S. (2015). Fluorescent porous carbon nanocapsules for two-photon imaging, NIR/pH dual-responsive drug carrier, and photothermal therapy. *Biomaterials*, **53**:117–126.

[24] Zhang H, Wu H, Wang J, Yang Y, Wu D, Zhang Y, Zhou Z and Yang S. (2015). Graphene oxide-BaGdF5 nanocomposites for multi-modal imaging and photothermal therapy. *Biomaterials*, **42**:66–77.

[25] Gollavelli G and Ling YC. (2014). Magnetic and fluorescent graphene for dual modal imaging and single light induced photothermal and photodynamic therapy of cancer cells. *Biomaterials*, **35**:4499–4507.

[26] Tao Y, Ju E, Ren J and Qu X. (2014). Immunostimulatory oligonucleotides-loaded cationic graphene oxide with photothermally enhanced immunogenicity for photothermal/immune cancer therapy. *Biomaterials*, **35**:9963–9971.

[27] Wang S, Zhang Q, Luo XF, Li J, He H, Yang F, Di Y, Jin C, Jiang XG, Shen S and Fu DL. (2014). Magnetic graphene-based nanotheranostic agent for dual-modality mapping guided photothermal therapy in regional lymph nodal metastasis of pancreatic cancer. *Biomaterials*, **35**:9473–9483.

[28] Lu YJ, Lin CW, Yang HW, Lin KJ, Wey SP, Sun CL, Wei KC, Yen TC, Lin CL, Ma CC and Chen JP. (2014). Biodistribution of PEGylated graphene oxide nanoribbons and their application in cancer chemo-photothermal therapy. *Carbon*, **74**:83–95.

[29] Sheng Z, Song L, Zheng J, Hu D, He M, Zheng M, Gao G, Gong P, Zhang P, Ma Y and Cai L. (2013). Protein-assisted fabrication of nano-reduced graphene oxide for combined *in vivo* photoacoustic imaging and photothermal therapy. *Biomaterials*, **34**:5236–5243.

[30] Shi X, Gong H, Li Y, Wang C, Cheng L and Liu Z. (2013). Graphene-based magnetic plasmonic nanocomposite for dual bioimaging and photothermal therapy. *Biomaterials*, **34**:4786–4793.

[31] Sahu A, Choi WI, Lee JH and Tae G. (2013). Graphene oxide mediated delivery of methylene blue for combined photodynamic and photothermal therapy. *Biomaterials*, **34**:6239–6248.

[32] Wang Y, Wang H, Liu D, Song S, Wang X and Zhang H. (2013). Graphene oxide covalently grafted upconversion nanoparticles for combined NIR mediated imaging and photothermal/photodynamic cancer therapy. *Biomaterials*, **34**:7715–7724.

[33] Wang L, Shi J, Zhang H, Li H, Gao Y, Wang Z, *et al.* (2013). Synergistic anticancer effect of RNAi and photothermal therapy mediated by functionalized single-walled carbon nanotubes. *Biomaterials*, **34**:262–274.

[34] Chu M, Peng J, Zhao J, Liang S, Shao Y and Wu Q. (2013). Laser light triggered-activated carbon nanosystem for cancer therapy. *Biomaterials*, **34**:1820–1832.

[35] Moon HK, Lee SH and Choi HC. (2009). *In vivo* near-infrared mediated tumor destruction by photothermal effect of carbon nanotubes. *ACS Nano*, **3**:3707–3713.

[36] Hashida Y, Tanaka H, Zhou S, Kawakami S, Yamashita F, Murakami T, Umeyama T, Imahori H and Hashida M. (2014). Photothermal ablation of

tumor cells using a single-walled carbon nanotube–peptide composite. *Journal of Controlled Release*. **173**:59–66.

[37] Zhang M, Murakami T, Ajima K, Tsuchida K, Sandanayaka AS, Ito O, Iijima S and Yudasaka M. (2008). Fabrication of ZnPc/protein nanohorns for double photodynamic and hyperthermic cancer phototherapy. *Proc. Natl. Acad. Sci. USA*, **105**:14773–14778.

[38] Whitney JR, Sarkar S, Zhang J, Do T, Young T, Manson MK, Campbell TA, Puretzky AA, Rouleau CM, More KL, Geohegan DB, Rylander CG, Dorn HC and Rylander MN. (2011). Single walled carbon nanohorns as photothermal cancer agents. *Lasers Surg. Med.*, **43**:43–51.

[39] Jung HS, Kong WH, Sung DK, Lee MY, Beack SE, Keum do H, Kim KS, Yun SH and Hahn SK. (2014). Nanographene oxide-hyaluronic acid conjugate for photothermal ablation therapy of skin cancer. *ACS Nano*, **8**:260–268.

[40] Yang K, Zhang S, Zhang G, Sun X, Lee ST and Liu Z. (2010). Graphene in mice: ultrahigh *in vivo* tumor uptake and efficient photothermal therapy. *Nano Lett*, **10**:3318–3323.

[41] Chen HW, Burnett J, Zhang FX, Zhang JM, Paholak H and Sun DX. (2014). Highly crystallized iron oxide nanoparticles as effective and biodegradable mediators for photothermal cancer therapy. *J. Mater. Chem. B,* **2**:757–765.

[42] Shen S, Kong F, Guo X, Wu L, Shen H, Xie M, Wang X, Jin Y and Ge Y. (2013). CMCTS stabilized Fe3O4 particles with extremely low toxicity as highly efficient near-infrared photothermal agents for *in vivo* tumor ablation. *Nanoscale*, **5**:8056–8066.

[43] Chu M, Shao Y, Peng J, Dai X, Li H, Wu Q and Shi D. (2013). Near-infrared laser light mediated cancer therapy by photothermal effect of Fe3O4 magnetic nanoparticles. *Biomaterials*, **34**:4078–4088.

[44] Liao MY, Lai PS, Yu HP, Lin HP and Huang CC. (2012). Innovative ligand-assisted synthesis of NIR-activated iron oxide for cancer theranostics. *Chem. Commun. (Camb)*, **48**:5319–5321.

[45] Yang K, Xu H, Cheng L, Sun C, Wang J and Liu Z. (2012). *In vitro* and *in vivo* near-infrared photothermal therapy of cancer using polypyrrole organic nanoparticles. *Adv. Mater.*, **24**:5586–5592.

[46] Cheng L, Yang K, Chen Q and Liu Z. (2012). Organic stealth nanoparticles for highly effective *in vivo* near-infrared photothermal therapy of cancer. *ACS Nano*, **6**:5605–5613.

[47] Zhou J, Lu Z, Zhu X, Wang X, Liao Y, Ma Z and Li F. (2013). NIR photothermal therapy using polyaniline nanoparticles. *Biomaterials*, **34**:9584–9592.

[48] Chu M, Li H, Wu Q, Wo F and Shi D. (2014). Pluronic-encapsulated natural chlorophyll nanocomposites for *in vivo* cancer imaging and photothermal/photodynamic therapies. *Biomaterials*, **35**:8357–8373.

[49] Goel S, Chen F and Cai W. (2014). Synthesis and biomedical applications of copper sulfide nanoparticles: from sensors to theranostics. *Small*, **10**:631–645.

[50] Liu X, Li B, Fu F, Xu K, Zou R, Wang Q, Zhang B, Chen Z and Hu J. (2014). Facile synthesis of biocompatible cysteine-coated CuS nanoparticles with high photothermal conversion efficiency for cancer therapy. *Dalton Trans.*, **43**:11709–11715.

[51] Li B, Wang Q, Zou R, Liu X, Xu K, Li W and Hu J. (2014). $Cu_{7.2}S_4$ nanocrystals: a novel photothermal agent with a 56.7% photothermal conversion efficiency for photothermal therapy of cancer cells. *Nanoscale*, **6**:3274–3282.

[52] Song GC, Wang Q, Wang Y, Lv G, Li C, Zou R, Chen ZG, Qin ZY, Huo K, Hu RG and Hu JQ. (2013). A Low-Toxic Multifunctional Nanoplatform Based on Cu9S5@mSiO2 Core-Shell Nanocomposites: Combining Photothermal- and Chemotherapies with Infrared Thermal Imaging for Cancer Treatment. *Nanoscale*, **23**:4281–4291.

[53] Tian Q, Hu J, Zhu Y, Zou R, Chen Z, Yang S, Li R , Su Q , Han Y and Liu X. (2013). Sub-10 nm Fe3O4@Cu(2-x)S core-shell nanoparticles for dual-modal imaging and photothermal therapy. *J. Am. Chem. Soc.*, **135**:8571–8577.

[54] Li W, Zamani R, Rivera Gil P, Pelaz B, Ibanez M, Cadavid D, Shavel A, Alvarez-Puebla RA, Parak WJ, Arbiol J and Cabot A. (2013). CuTe nanocrystals: shape and size control, plasmonic properties, and use as SERS probes and photothermal agents. *J. Am. Chem. Soc.*, **135**:7098–7101.

[55] Chu M, Pan X, Zhang D, Wu Q, Peng J and Hai W. (2012). The therapeutic efficacy of CdTe and CdSe quantum dots for photothermal cancer therapy. *Biomaterials*, **33**:7071–7083.

[56] Tian Q, Tang M, Sun Y, Zou R, Chen Z, Zhu M, Yang S, Wang J, Wang J and Hu J. (2011). Hydrophilic flower-like CuS superstructures as an efficient 980 nm laser-driven photothermal agent for ablation of cancer cells. *Adv. Mater.*, **23**:3542–3547.

[57] Hessel CM, Pattani VP, Rasch M, Panthani MG, Koo B, Tunnell JW and Korgel BA. (2011). Copper selenide nanocrystals for photothermal therapy. *Nano Lett.*, **11**:2560–2566.

[58] Tian Q, Jiang F, Zou R, Liu Q, Chen Z, Zhu M, *et al.* (2011). Hydrophilic Cu_9S_5 nanocrystals: a photothermal agent with a 25.7% heat conversion efficiency for photothermal ablation of cancer cells *in vivo*. *ACS Nano*, **5**:9761–9771.

[59] Li Y, Lu W, Huang Q, Huang M, Li C and Chen W. (2010). Copper sulfide nanoparticles for photothermal ablation of tumor cells. *Nanomedicine (Lond)*, **5**:1161–1171.

[60] Choi HS, Liu W, Misra P, Tanaka E, Zimmer JP, Itty Ipe B, Bawendi MG and Frangioni JV. (2007). Renal clearance of quantum dots. *Nat. Biotechnol.*, **25**:1165–1170.

[61] Jiang W, Kim BY, Rutka JT and Chan WC. (2008). Nanoparticle-mediated cellular response is size-dependent. *Nat. Nanotechnol.*, **3**:145–150.

[62] Gao H, Shi W and Freund LB. (2005). Mechanics of receptor-mediated endocytosis. *Proc. Natl. Acad. Sci. USA*, **102**:9469–9474.

[63] Zhu YD, Peng J, Jiang LP and Zhu JJ. (2014). Fluorescent immunosensor based on CuS nanoparticles for sensitive detection of cancer biomarker. *Analyst.*, **139**:649–655.

[64] Cheng CY, Ou KL, Huang WT, Chen JK, Chang JY and Yang CH. (2013). Gadolinium-based CuInS2/ZnS nanoprobe for dual-modality magnetic resonance/optical imaging. *ACS Appl. Mater. Interfaces*, **5**:4389–4400.

[65] Pons T, Pic E, Lequeux N, Cassette E, Bezdetnaya L, Guillemin F, Marchal F and Dubertret B. (2010). Cadmium-free CuInS2/ZnS quantum dots for sentinel lymph node imaging with reduced toxicity. *ACS Nano*, **4**:2531–2538.

[66] Ku G, Zhou M, Song S, Huang Q, Hazle J and Li C. (2012). Copper sulfide nanoparticles as a new class of photoacoustic contrast agent for deep tissue imaging at 1064 nm. *ACS Nano*, **6**:7489–7496.

[67] Zhao Y, Pan H, Lou Y, Qiu X, Zhu J and Burda C. (2009). Plasmonic Cu(2-x)S nanocrystals: optical and structural properties of copper-deficient copper(I) sulfides. *J. Am. Chem. Soc.*, **131**:4253–4261.

[68] Bayliss SC, Heald R, Fletcher DI and Buckberry LD. (1999). The culture of mammalian cells on nanostructured silicon. *Adv. Mater.*, **11**:318–321.

[69] Canham LT. (1995). Bioactive silicon structure fabrication through nanoetching techniques. *Adv. Mater.*, **7**:1033–1037.

[70] Park JH, Gu L, von Maltzahn G, Ruoslahti E, Bhatia SN and Sailor MJ. (2009). Biodegradable luminescent porous silicon nanoparticles for *in vivo* applications. *Nat. Mater.*, **8**:331–336.

[71] Ma YF, Li Y and Zhong XH. (2014). Silica coating of luminescent quantum dots prepared in aqueous media for cellular labeling. *Journal of Nanoparticle Research*, **60**:543–551.

[72] Chu MQ, Sun Y and Xu S. (2008). Silica-coated quantum dots fluorescent spheres synthesized using a quaternary 'water-in-oil' microemulsion system. *Journal of Nanoparticle Research*, **10**:613–624.

[73] Camerin M, Magaraggia M, Soncin M, Jori G, Moreno M, Chambrier I, Cook MJ and Russell DA. (2010). The *in vivo* efficacy of phthalocyanine-nanoparticle conjugates for the photodynamic therapy of amelanotic melanoma. *Eur. J. Cancer*, **46**:1910–1918.

[74] Borgul O and Kaplan M. (2012). Photodynamic therapy of dermal metastases of disseminated melanoma. *Photodiagn Photodyn. Ther.*, **9**:9–10.

[75] Kawczyk-Krupka A, Bugaj AM, Latos W, Zaremba K and Sieron A. (2013). Photodynamic therapy in treatment of cutaneous and choroidal melanoma. *Photodiagnosis Photodyn. Ther.*, **10**:503–509.

Chapter 7

Semiconductor Quantum Dot-tagged Graphene Nanosheets for Bioimaging and Cancer Dual Modal Therapy

Developing nanomaterials with multiple functions and low toxicity is currently one of the research goals in nanobiomedicine. Hybrid nanocomposites composed of semiconductor quantum dots (QDs) and graphene nanosheets are novel multifunctional nanomaterials that can be used for cancer fluorescence imaging, and photothermal and photodynamic cancer therapy. Graphene oxide (GO) and reduced graphene oxide (rGO) are the most popular types of graphene nanosheets used in biomedical research. Toxic metal cations, like cadmium ions, and drugs, such as doxorubicin, may be strongly adsorbed by GO and rGO. Therefore, the toxicity of QDs is lowered by combination with graphene nanosheets because the toxic metal ions released from the QDs are captured by the nanosheets. In addition, a large amount of drugs can be loaded onto QD-GO/rGO nanocomposites. Such drug-loaded QD-GO/rGO nanocomposites may exhibit the synergistic effects of drug therapy (e.g., chemotherapy), and photothermal and photodynamic therapies. In this Chapter, the advantages of combining QDs with graphene nanosheets, bioimaging and cancer therapy using QD-GO/rGO nanocomposites and their preparation are discussed. The disadvantages of QD-GO/rGO nanocomposites such as low fluorescence quantum yield are also described.

1. Introduction

In recent years, semiconductor QDs have been combined with many interesting organic and inorganic materials to lower the toxicity of QDs, improve their properties and generate novel multifunctional nanocomposites. For example, Jun *et al.* [1] deposited core–shell QDs composed of a cadmium selenide (CdSe) core and cadmium sulfide (CdS) shell onto the surface of silica (SiO_2) nanoparticles with a diameter of approximately 120 nm, and then encapsulated the SiO_2/QD nanocomposites with a SiO_2 shell. The resulting material was not only less toxic than the equivalent number of SiO_2-free single QDs, but also exhibited 200-fold stronger photoluminescence emission than single QDs. In another example, Jin and co-workers coated CdSe/zinc sulfide (ZnS) QDs with a gold (Au) nanoshell [2]. In their experiments, the hydrophobic CdSe/ZnS QDs were coated with a lipid–polyethylene glycol (PEG)–COOH layer and then poly-L-histidine (PLH) to immobilize a high density of Au^{3+} ions. After addition of hydroxylamine, a thin Au shell was formed on the PLH template. The spacing between the QD core and Au shell was controlled by the thickness of the lipid-PEG–COOH layer. The QD-Au core–shell nanocomposites exhibited strong fluorescence, allowing them to be used as probes for surface plasmon scattering. The gold shell not only lowered the toxicity of the QDs, but also facilitated functionalization of the nanocomposite.

Graphene is a sp^2-bonded carbon nanosheet with a hexagonal lattice with one atom at each vertex. An ideal graphene nanosheet has only a single atomic layer of carbon. This two-dimensional carbon nanomaterial is a basic building block for graphitic materials of all other dimensionalities, like fullerenes (zero-dimensional), carbon nanotubes (one-dimensional) and graphite (three-dimensional) (Fig. 7.1) [3]. Geim and Novoselov won the Nobel Prize in Physics in 2010 for their groundbreaking experiments on graphene [4]. Since then, this allotrope of carbon has captivated many scientists globally because it has a large specific surface area, and exhibits interesting mechanical, electrical, optical, thermal and chemical properties. In biomedical research, graphene nanosheets have been used for drug and gene delivery [5–7], bioimaging [8, 9], biosensing [10, 11],

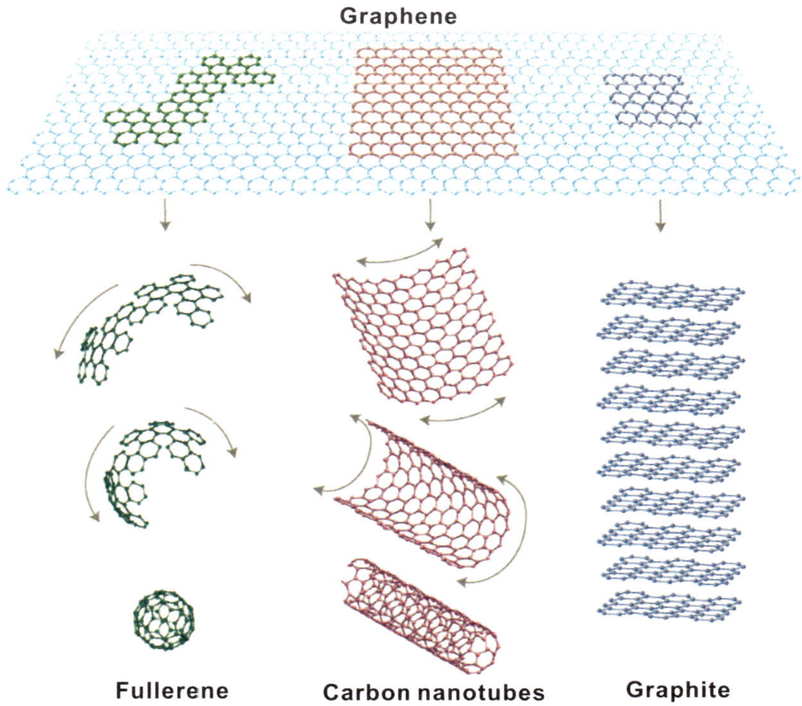

Fig. 7.1. Graphene nanosheet is the precursor to generate all graphitic carbon materials. Reprinted with permission from Ref. [3]. Copyright (2007) Nature Publishing Group.

cancer photothermal therapy (PTT) [12, 13] and tissue engineering [14, 15]. When QDs are incorporated into graphene nanosheets, the resulting nanocomposites are less toxic and possess more functions than the QDs alone.

2. Advantages of Combining Semiconductor QDs with Graphene Nanosheets

2.1 Reducing the toxicity of QDs

Water-soluble graphene oxide (GO) and reduced graphene oxide (rGO) have ultra-high ratios of surface area to volume and many negative charges. Therefore, GO and rGO nanosheets can strongly adsorb positive ions, as well as drugs. For example, the adsorption capacities of GO and rGO for lead(II) cations are 30 and 15 mg/g, respectively [16]. These graphene derivatives can also adsorb metal cations like copper(II) (Cu^{2+}), cadmium(II) (Cd^{2+}), mercury(II), iron(II), cobalt(II), nickel(II), and chromium(VI) through the strong affinity between graphene and metal ions [16–19].

Semiconductor QDs are usually made of heavy metal ions such as Cd^{2+} and Cu^{2+}. The toxicity of QDs mainly caused by the release of these heavy ions from the QDs. Because graphene nanosheets can adsorb these toxic positive ions, QD-graphene nanocomposites may exhibit lower toxicity than the QDs alone. In addition, the stabilizers capped on the surfaces of QDs such as mercaptopropionic acid (MPA) are also highly toxic to cells and animals. Conjugation of stabilizer-capped QDs to rGO may decrease the opportunity for direct contact between the toxic stabilizer and cells, and rGO may also adsorb these stabilizers. For example, our research group [20] recently modified copper indium sulfide ($CuInS_2$)/ZnS core–shell QDs with lipid bilayers and 1,2-distearoyl-sn-glycero-3-phosphoethanolamine-N-(amino[polyethylene glycol]-2000) (DSPE-PEG_{2000}-NH_2), and then conjugated them with rGO via covalent bonding (Fig. 7.2). The liposome-coated $CuInS_2$/ZnS QDs and $CuInS_2$/ZnS QD-tagged rGO were then injected into tumor-bearing mice. The mass of Cu^{2+} ions in the tumors of

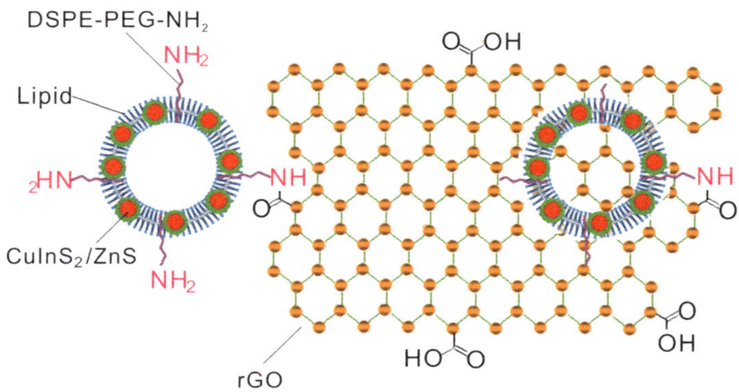

Fig. 7.2. Schematic illustration of the structure of a $CuInS_2$/ZnS-tagged rGO nanocomposite.

the $CuInS_2$/ZnS QD group 7, 30 and 60 days after injection were always obviously lower than that of Cu^{2+} ions in the tumors of the $CuInS_2$/ZnS QD-tagged rGO group examined at the same time points. In addition, the main organs such as the liver of mice in the $CuInS_2$/ZnS QD-tagged rGO group contained a lower concentration of Cu^{2+} ions than those in the $CuInS_2$/ZnS QD group. This indicated that some Cu^{2+} ions released from the QDs may strongly bind to rGO, so rGO delayed the migration of Cu^{2+} ions into deep organs of the mice injected with $CuInS_2$/ZnS QD-tagged rGO. When human esophageal squamous carcinoma cells (Eca-109) were incubated with the liposome-coated $CuInS_2$/ZnS QDs and $CuInS_2$/ZnS QD-tagged rGO, the cell viability in the $CuInS_2$/ZnS QD group was much lower than that in the $CuInS_2$/ZnS QD-tagged rGO group. For example, nearly all cells died after they were incubated with the liposome-coated $CuInS_2$/ZnS QDs (10 μg/mL) for 72 h, whereas 46.96 ± 11.90% of cells survived that were incubated with the liposome-coated $CuInS_2$/ZnS QD-tagged rGO (containing 10 μg/mL of $CuInS_2$/ZnS QDs) for 72 h.

In 2012, Hu *et al.* [21] conjugated 11-mercaptoundecanoic acid (MUA)- or MPA-capped CdSe/ZnS QDs onto rGO and also demonstrated that QD toxicity could be substantially reduced by the conjugation of rGO. They found that when human carcinoma (HeLa) and MCF-7 cancer cells were incubated with 20 mg/L QD-rGO for 12 to 48 h, most of the cells (~92%) survived. In contrast, cell viabilities significantly decreased when they were incubated with MUA- and MPA-capped QDs without rGO, respectively.

2.2 Exhibiting multiple functionalities

Single nanosystems that exhibit multiple functionalities have attracted much attention in nanobiomedical research because they have great potential for clinic applications. QDs possess outstanding optical properties that have been widely used in biomedical imaging and cancer therapy. Meanwhile, graphene nanosheets are excellent drug carriers and photothermal agents. Therefore, the nanocomposites obtained by combining QDs and rGO may display various biofunctions.

To produce QD-rGO nanomaterials with high fluorescent quantum yield, a suitable size of rGO should be selected. In general, QD fluorescence is easily quenched or shielded by large-sized rGO. For example, when poly(l-lysine)-modified CdSe/ZnS QDs were deposited onto micrometer-sized rGO surfaces, no fluorescent signal was detected [21]. However, when the size of rGO was decreased to about 260 and 38 nm, the corresponding QD-rGO composites displayed fluorescence that was 50% and 85%, respectively, as intense as that of the QDs alone. This behavior may be related to the radiation-shielding effect of larger rGO sheets and energy transfer from the QDs to rGO. Therefore, after the CdSe/ZnS QDs were combined with ultra-small rGO, the resulting CdSe/ZnS-rGO nanocomposite emitted bright QD fluorescence. When CdSe/ZnS QD-rGO materials that exhibited green and red fluorescence were subcutaneously injected (~2 mm deep) into a mouse, their bright fluorescence was clearly observed.

Because the QDs deposited on small-sized rGO retain their fluorescence, the interaction between QD-rGO bioconjugates and cancer cells may be conveniently observed through fluorescence imaging. When a CdSe/ZnS QD-rGO nanocomposite was conjugated with folic acid (FA) and then incubated with FA receptor-expressing MCF-7 and HeLa cells, the nanocomposite particles in or on cells could be observed under a fluorescence microscope [21]. For example, QD-rGO-FA with smaller-sized rGO (~38 nm) could penetrate into cancer cells, whereas QD-rGO-FA with larger-sized rGO (~260 nm) was mainly located on cell surfaces. In addition, QD-rGO-FA with smaller-sized rGO was found in many regions of the cytoplasm.

Besides fluorescence imaging, QD-rGO nanocomposites can also kill cancer cells upon laser irradiation. Furthermore, intracellular nanocomposites may be more efficient at killing cells than extracellular ones. For example, when MCF-7 cells were incubated with QD-rGO-FA with smaller-sized rGO (~38 nm, QDs in 20 mg/cm, in terms of the rGO amount) for 24 h and then irradiated with an 808 nm laser (2 W/cm^2) for 9 min, only 5% of the cells survived. However, when QD-rGO-FA with larger rGO (~260 nm) was incubated with MCF-7 cells under the same conditions, more than 30% of the cells survived. This is because the smaller QD-rGO-FA nanocomposite migrated into cells via FA receptor-mediated endocytosis, whereas most of the larger QD-rGO-FA nanocomposite was not easily taken up by the cells.

Graphene nanosheets can load drugs by π–π stacking, hydrogen bonding, electrostatic and hydrophobic interactions. It has been demonstrated that 100 mg of GO could be loaded with 186.6 mg of doxorubicin (DOX) at pH = 6.5, a chemotherapy drug, and could be loaded with 382.7 mg of DOX at pH = 8.0 [22]. GO can also synchronously load different kinds of drugs. For example, the loading efficiencies of photosensitizer chlorin e6 and DOX onto PEG-grafted GO nanosheets were 51.9 ± 5.1% and 61.7 ± 4.4%, respectively [23]. Therefore, QD-rGO nanocomposites have great potential to load drugs for multimodal therapy. If chemotherapy drugs and/or photosensitizers are incorporated into QD-rGO nanocomposites, the efficiency of cancer therapy using the drug-loaded QD-rGO nanocomposite may be considerably improved compared with that using the drug(s) and nanocomposite alone.

2.3 Improving the efficiency of cancer phototherapy

In previous chapters, it has been mentioned that upon red or laser irradiation, QD can not only convert light energy into heat, but also generate intracellular reactive oxygen species (ROS). This means that QDs without additional photosensitizers can be used for both PTT and photodynamic therapy (PDT) to treat cancer. Our research group [20] detected the photothermal conversion efficiency and intracellular ROS level of liposome-coated $CuInS_2/ZnS$ QDs after laser irradiation. The temperature of solutions of the $CuInS_2/ZnS$ QDs (200 μL, 0.05 and 0.5 mg/mL) increased by 18 and 30°C, respectively, after 20 min of 671 nm laser irradiation at a power density of 0.2 W/cm^2. We also found that the temperatures of solutions of rGO with the same concentrations as those of the $CuInS_2/ZnS$ QD ones were 5–15°C higher than the QD solutions when both were irradiated at 671 nm for 20 min. The intracellular ROS levels of $CuInS_2/ZnS$ QD solutions with concentrations of 5, 25, and 50 μg/mL following 20 min of 671 nm laser irradiation were 4.65 ± 0.77, 7.43 ± 1.19, 10.53 ± 0.94 times higher, respectively, than that of the untreated control cells. However, the level of ROS generated by rGO was significant lower than that generated by the QDs.

The above results suggest that QD-rGO nanocomposites may exhibit high ROS generation because of the QDs and strong photothermal conversion originating from rGO. That is to say, QD-rGO nanocomposites may show higher efficacy of cancer therapy than the QDs and rGO alone because of synergistic photothermal and photodynamic effects. Although both liposome-coated $CuInS_2$/ZnS QDs and rGO could kill Eca-109 cells upon 671 nm laser irradiation, $CuInS_2$/ZnS QD-tagged rGO killed the cancer cells much more effectively than either the QDs or rGO alone [20]. For example [20], when Eca-109 cells were incubated with $CuInS_2$/ZnS QD-tagged rGO containing 0.25 mg/mL of $CuInS_2$/ZnS QDs and 0.05 mg/mL of rGO and irradiated at 671 nm laser for 20 min, all cancer cells died. In contrast, $30.97 \pm 24.43\%$ and $52.43 \pm 8.41\%$ of cells survived when they were incubated with 0.25 mg/mL of $CuInS_2$/ZnS QDs and 0.05 mg/mL of rGO, respectively, and then irradiated at 671 nm for 20 min. The stabilizers on the QD surfaces had no toxicity to cells in these experiments because they were liposomes.

The high phototherapeutic efficacy of QD-rGO nanocomposites was also demonstrated in animal experiments. For example [20], when 50 μL of a solution of $CuInS_2$/ZnS QD-tagged rGO containing 2.5 mg/mL of $CuInS_2$/ZnS QDs and 0.5 mg/mL of rGO was intratumorally injected into mice with tumors grown from Eca-109 cells and irradiated by a 671 nm laser for 20 min each day, all mouse tumors (n=6) disappeared after 18 days of irradiation. In contrast, the tumors that were injected with QDs or rGO (n=6 for each group) and irradiated with at 671 nm for 20 min each day for 18 days did not completely disappear. Such QD-rGO nanocomposites with low toxicity, bright fluorescence and highly efficacious cancer PTT and PDT may be interesting for both materials scientists and clinicians.

3. Preparation of Semiconductor QD-tagged Graphene Nanosheets

To date, QDs composed of CdS [24–26], CdSe [27], CdSe/ZnS [21, 28], CdTe [29–32], ZnS [33, 34], lead sulfide [35, 36], ZnO [37], cobalt sulfide [38], cobalt oxide [39], $CuInS_2$ [40], and $CuInS_2$/ZnS [20], etc., have been incorporated into graphene nanosheets. The methods used to prepare these

QD-graphene nanocomposites include *in situ* synthesis, electrostatic interaction or assembly and covalent reaction. Most QD-graphene nanocomposites have been prepared for optoelectronics or sensor applications. Only several groups have investigated the biomedical applications of QD-graphene nanocomposites.

The most popular method used to prepare QD-graphene nanocomposites is *in situ* synthesis. In this approach, graphene nanosheets act as a nucleation matrix for QDs or the supporting matrix for the crystal nuclei of QDs. As a result, the final QDs are directly adsorbed onto the graphene nanosheets, so no extra molecular linkers are required to combine the QDs and graphene. In 2010, Cao *et al.* [24] developed a one-step method to synthesize CdS-graphene using GO, cadmium acetate ($Cd(CH_3COO)_2$) and dimethyl sulfoxide (DMSO) as precursors. Cao and colleagues dispersed GO and $Cd(CH_3COO)_2{\bullet}2H_2O$ in DMSO, and then heated the mixture at 180°C for 12 h. After being washed with acetone and alcohol, the product could be resuspended in different solvents by sonication. The CdS QDs on the graphene sheets were 10 nm in diameter with blende structure. Nearly all graphene sheets were decorated with CdS nanoparticles, and the individual CdS QDs were well separated from each other. DMSO plays important roles during the formation of this CdS-graphene nanocomposite. At 180°C, DMSO provides the reductant hydrogen sulfide that reacts with $Cd(CH_3COO)_2$, and DMSO also reduces GO sheets to graphene. Therefore, this method involves the simultaneous reduction of GO sheets to graphene and formation of CdS QDs.

In 2011, Lu *et al.* [31] developed a more rapid and environmentally friendly method to prepare QD-graphene nanocomposites. They replaced DMSO with water and then mixed 1-thioglycerol-coated CdTe QDs and GO in water to form hydrogen bonds between 1-thioglycerol on the surface of the CdTe and GO. The mixture was heated at 200°C for just 45 min. During this process, the GO sheets were reduced to graphene, and the CdTe on the graphene surface grew larger (Fig. 7.3). Both AFM and TEM images confirmed the attachment of CdTe to the graphene nanosheets (Fig. 7.4). This is also an one-step *in situ* synthesis method, because both the reduction of GO to graphene and growth of QDs on graphene occurred simultaneously during the hydrothermal reaction.

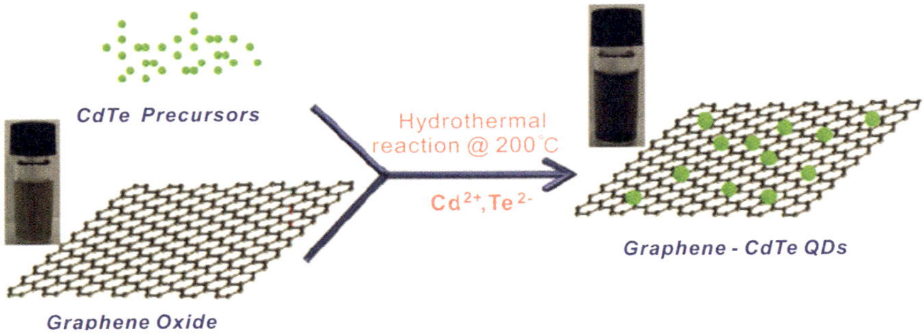

Fig. 7.3. Schematic illustration of the preparation of CdTe-graphene nanocomposites through one-step hydrothermal reaction. Reprinted with permission from Ref. [31]. Copyright (2010) Elsevier.

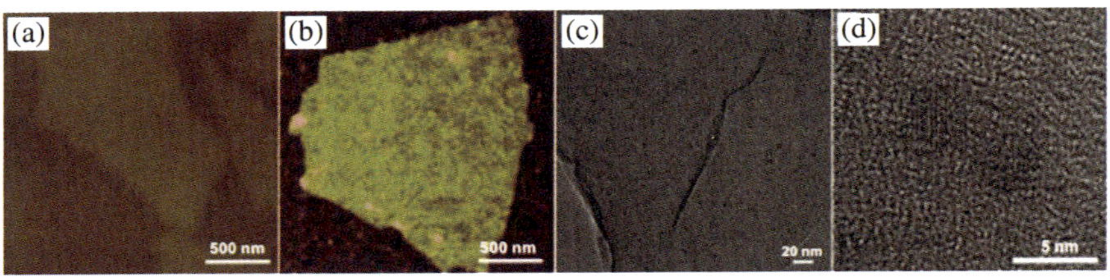

Fig. 7.4. AFM and TEM images of graphene and a CdTe-graphene nanocomposite. AFM images of (a) graphene nanosheets and (b) CdTe-graphene nanocomposite. (c) TEM and (d) high-resolution TEM images of the CdTe-graphene nanocomposite. Reprinted with permission from Ref. [31]. Copyright (2010) Elsevier.

QD-graphene nanocomposites can also be prepared by electrophoretic deposition. In 2015, Sun *et al.* [37] used this method to synthesize ZnO QD-graphene composites with an electrophoretic deposition device (Fig. 7.5a). To prepare the ZnO-graphene composites, they positioned electrodes patterned with graphene into a solution of $Zn(CH_3COO)_2{\cdot}2H_2O$ in ethanol at 0°C, and then added an ethanol solution of lithium hydroxide monohydrate. After 1 h, the substrate was washed and then dried under nitrogen atmosphere. The product consisted of spherical ZnO nanoparticles with a diameter of ~6 nm uniformly attached to the surface of graphene sheets (Fig. 7.5b).

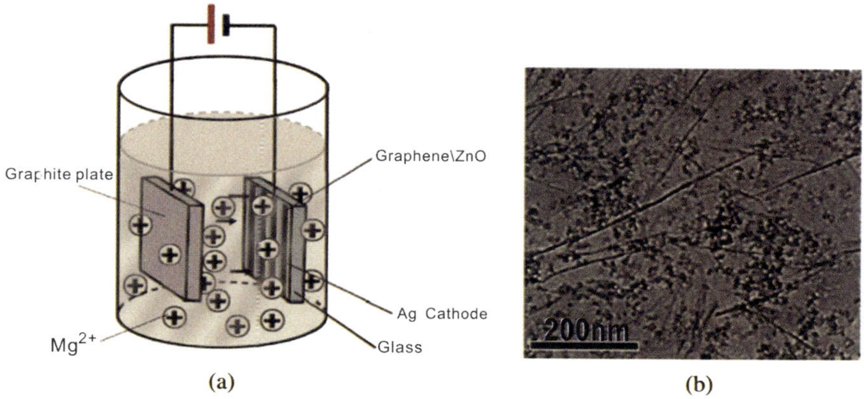

Fig. 7.5. Preparation of a ZnO-graphene nanocomposite. (a) Schematic illustration of electrophoretic deposition. (b) TEM image of the ZnO-graphene nanocomposite. Reprinted with permission from Ref. [37]. Copyright (2015) Elsevier.

The QD-graphene nanocomposites prepared by the methods described above have no or low fluorescence because it is quenched by graphene. Therefore, these QD-graphene composites may be used for cancer phototherapy, but may be not suitable for bioimaging. To overcome this limitation, QDs on graphene surfaces should be protected by a shell and the distance between the QDs and graphene should be increased.

To prepare QD-graphene composites that emit strong fluorescence, the surfaces of both the QDs and graphene should be modified before their combination. In 2011, Chen *et al.* [32] developed fluorescent QD-graphene conjugates for *in vitro* imaging of live HeLa cells. In Chen and co-workers' experiments, GO sheets were reduced to rGO by poly(sodium 4-styrenesulfonate) (PSS) at 100°C, and then coated with polyethylenimine (PEI) via the electrostatic interaction between PSS and PEI. At the same time, thioglycolic acid-capped CdTe QDs were coated with bovine serum albumin (BSA) through the formation of amide bonds. CdTe-rGO nanocomposites were then obtained by mixing the PEI/PSS-coated rGO and BSA-coated CdTe. CdTe QDs could be strongly adsorbed by rGO via the negatively charged amino acid residues on the surface of the BSA-coated CdTe and the cationic groups of the outer layer of polyelectrolyte deposited on the rGO. Compared with uncoated CdTe, the CdTe-rGO composites exhibited strong absorption from ultraviolet to NIR regions. The fluorescence emission of the BSA-coated QDs on PEI/PSS-coated rGO was more intense than that of the uncoated QDs on the modified rGO. This is because the surface defects of the uncoated CdTe QDs may have been passivated by the polymers, and rGO cannot significantly quench the QD fluorescence because they are both protected by polymers. These CdTe-rGO nanocomposites with bright fluorescence can be used for cancer cell labeling and imaging because the BSA molecules on the CdTe-rGO surface can interact with cellular membranes and be taken up by cancer cells, even in the absence of specific targeting molecules.

Hu and colleagues also prepared highly fluorescent QD-graphene nanocomposites [21]. They coated rGO with amphiphilic polypeptide poly(l-lysine) and CdSe/ZnS QDs with MUA. The positively charged CdSe/ZnS were readily adsorbed onto the polypeptide-coated rGO, and the resulting QD-rGO nanocomposite displayed bright fluorescence. Recently, our research group [20] prepared $CuInS_2$/ZnS-tagged rGO via covalent reaction (see Fig. 7.2 above). Because the $CuInS_2$/ZnS-tagged rGO exhibited bright red fluorescence, these nanocomposites could be used for *in vivo* imaging.

4. Discussion

Although QD-tagged graphene nanosheets have many advantages compared with QDs and graphene nanosheets alone as described above, these nanocomposites also have many limitations. First, the quantum yield of QD fluorescence decreases substantially after being incorporated into graphene nanosheets, particularly if the distance between them is less than 10 nm. Coating the QDs with a polymer or SiO_2 shell can prevent quenching of QD fluorescence. However, the fluorescence of polymer- or SiO_2-coated QDs may still be reduced by the graphene nanosheets because polymer and SiO_2 shells are usually porous. In addition, the fluorescence quantum yield of QDs depends strongly on the size of the graphene nanosheets used in the nanocomposites [21]. The excitation or emission of QDs can be shielded by large sheets. For example, the fluorescence of QDs deposited onto micrometer-sized graphene nanosheets was difficult to detect [21]. Second, the ability of graphene nanosheets to adsorb the toxic metal ions released from QDs is limited. Several nanometer-sized semiconductor QDs contain thousands of metal ions. Once the graphene nanosheets are saturated with adsorbed metal ions, any further metal ions leaked from the QDs would migrate into nearby cells. Therefore, the ability of graphene nanosheets to lower QD toxicity should be improved. Third, the dispersion of QD-graphene nanosheet composites in aqueous solution is poorer than that of QDs and graphene alone. These limitations need to be overcome to facilitate the future use of such nanocomposites in cancer imaging and therapy.

References

[1] Jun BH, Hwang DW, Jung HS, Jang J, Kim H, Kang H, Kang T, Kyeong S, Lee H, Jeong DH, Kang KW, Youn H, Lee DS and Lee Y-S. (2012). Ultrasensitive, biocompatible, quantum-dot-embedded silica nanoparticles for bioimaging. *Adv. Funct. Mater.* **22**:1843–1849.

[2] Jin YD and Gao XH. (2009). Plasmonic fluorescent quantum dots. *Nat. Nanotechnol.*, **4**:571–576.

[3] Geim AK and Novoselov KS. (2007). The rise of graphene. *Nat. Mater.*, **6**:183–191.

[4] The Nobel Prize in Physics 2010. The Nobel Foundation. Retrieved 3 December 2013.

[5] Chen JQ, Liu HY, Zhao CB, Qin GQ, Xi GN, Li T, Wang XP and Chen TS. (2014). One-step reduction and PEGylation of graphene oxide for photothermally controlled drug delivery. *Biomaterials*, **35**:4986–4995.

[6] Miao W, Shim G, Kang CM, Lee S, Choe YS, Choi HG and Oh YK. (2013). Cholesteryl hyaluronic acid-coated, reduced graphene oxide nanosheets for anti-cancer drug delivery. *Biomaterials*, **34**:9638–9647.

[7] Liu JQ, Cui L and Losic D. (2013). Graphene and graphene oxide as new nanocarriers for drug delivery applications. *Acta Biomater*, **9**:9243–9257.

[8] Gollavelli G and Ling YC. (2012). Multi-functional graphene as an *in vitro* and *in vivo* imaging probe. *Biomaterials*, **33**:2532–2545.

[9] Sheng ZH, Song L, Zheng JX, Hu DH, He M, Zheng MB, Gao GH, Gong P, Zhang PF, Ma YF and Cai LT. (2013). Protein-assisted fabrication of nano-reduced graphene oxide for combined *in vivo* photoacoustic imaging and photothermal therapy. *Biomaterials*, **34**:5236–5243.

[10] Wang F, Zhu LH and Zhang JD. (2014). Electrochemical sensor for levofloxacin based on molecularly imprinted polypyrrole-graphene-gold nanoparticles modified electrode. *Sensor Actuat B-Chem.*, **192**:642–647.

[11] Artiles MS, Rout CS and Fisher TS. (2011). Graphene-based hybrid materials and devices for biosensing. *Adv. Drug Deliver Rev.*, **63**:1352–1360.

[12] Zhang W, Guo ZY, Huang DQ, Liu ZM, Guo X and Zhong HQ. (2011). Synergistic effect of chemo-photothermal therapy using PEGylated graphene oxide. *Biomaterials*, **32**:8555–8561.

[13] Yang K, Wan JM, Zhang S, Tian B, Zhang YJ and Liu Z. (2012). The influence of surface chemistry and size of nanoscale graphene oxide on photothermal therapy of cancer using ultra-low laser power. *Biomaterials*, **33**:2206–2214.

[14] Tian HC, Liu JQ, Wei DX, Kang XY, Zhang C, Du JC, Yang B, Chen X, Zhu HY, Nuli YN and Yang CS. (2014). Graphene oxide doped conducting polymer nanocomposite film for electrode-tissue interface. *Biomaterials*, **35**:2120–2129.

[15] Sayyar S, Murray E, Thompson BC, Gambhir S, Officer DL and Wallace GG. (2013). Covalently linked biocompatible graphene/polycaprolactone composites for tissue engineering. *Carbon*, **52**:296–304.

[16] Dong ZH, Zhang F, Wang D, Liu X and Jin J. (2015). Polydopamine-mediated surface-functionalization of graphene oxide for heavy metal ions removal. *J. Solid State Chem.*, **224**:88–93.

[17] Wang DY, Wang DW, Chen HA, Chen TR, Li SS, Yeh YC, Kuo TR, Liao JH, Chang YC, Chen WT, Wu SH, Hu CC, Chen CW and Chen CC. (2015). Photoluminescence quenching of graphene oxide by metal ions in aqueous media. *Carbon*, **82**:24–30.

[18] Dubey R BJ and Bajpai AK. (2015). Green synthesis of graphene sand composite (GSC) as novel adsorbentfor efficient removal of Cr (VI) ions from aqueous solution. *J. Water Process Eng.*, **5**:11.

[19] Hu XJ, Liu YG, Zeng GM, Wang H, You SH, Hu X, Tan XF, Chen AW and Guo FY. (2015). Effects of inorganic electrolyte anions on enrichment of Cu(II) ions with aminated Fe3O4/graphene oxide: Cu(II) speciation prediction and surface charge measurement. *Chemosphere*, **127**:35–41.

[20] Wu Q, Chu MQ, Shao YX, Wo FJ and Shi DL. (2016). Reduced graphene oxide conjugated with CuInS2/ZnS nanocrystals with low toxicity for enhanced photothermal and photodynamic cancer therapies. *Carbon*, **108**: 21–37.

[21] Hu SH, Chen YW, Hung WT, Chen IW and Chen SY. (2012). Quantum-dot-tagged reduced graphene oxide nanocomposites for bright fluorescence bioimaging and photothermal therapy monitored *in situ*. *Adv. Mater.*, **24**:1748–1754.

[22] Zhang Q, Li WW, Kong T, Su RG, Li N, Song Q, Tang ML, Liu LW and Cheng GS. (2013). Tailoring the interlayer interaction between doxorubicin-loaded graphene oxide nanosheets by controlling the drug content. *Carbon*, **51**:164–172.

[23] Miao W, Shim G, Lee S, Lee S, Choe YS and Oh YK. (2013). Safety and tumor tissue accumulation of pegylated graphene oxide nanosheets for co-delivery of anticancer drug and photosensitizer. *Biomaterials*, **34**:3402–3410.

[24] Cao AN, Liu Z, Chu SS, Wu MH, Ye ZM, Cai ZW, Chang YL, Wang SF, Gong QH and Liu YF. (2010). A Facile One-step method to produce graphene-CdS quantum dot nanocomposites as promising optoelectronic materials. *Adv Mater.*, **22**:103.

[25] Yang MH, Javadi A and Gong SQ. (2011). Sensitive electrochemical i最终 mmunosensor for the detection of cancer biomarker using quantum dot functionalized graphene sheets as labels. *Sensor Actuat B-Chem.*, **155**:357–360.

[26] Zhang XY, Xu F, Zhao BQ, Ji X, Yao YW, Wu DP, Gao ZY and Jiang K. (2014). Synthesis of CdS quantum dots decorated graphene nanosheets and non-enzymatic photoelectrochemical detection of glucose. *Electrochim Acta.*, **133**:615–622.

[27] Kanodarwala FK, Wang F, Reece PJ and Stride JA. (2014). Deposition of CdSe quantum dots on graphene sheets. *J. Lumin.*, **146**:46–52.

[28] Zhou ZM, Zhou J, Chen J, Yu RN, Zhang MZ, Song JT and Zhao YD. (2014). Carcino-embryonic antigen detection based on fluorescence resonance energy transfer between quantum dots and graphene oxide. *Biosens. Bioelectron.*, **59**:397–403.

[29] Alibolandi M, Hadizadeh F, Vajhedin F, Abnous K and Ramezani M. (2015). Design and fabrication of an aptasensor for chloramphenicol based on energy transfer of CdTe quantum dots to graphene oxide sheet. *Mat. Sci. Eng. C-Mater.*, **48**:611–619.

[30] Zhang CY, Wang L, Wang AM, Zhang SY, Mao CJ, Song JM, Niu HL, Jin BK and Tian YP. (2014). A novel electrochemiluminescence sensor based on nitrogen-doped graphene/CdTe quantum dots composite. *Appl. Surf. Sci.*, **315**:22–27.

[31] Lu ZS, Guo CX, Yang HB, Qiao Y, Guo J and Li CM. (2011). One-step aqueous synthesis of graphene-CdTe quantum dot-composed nanosheet and its enhanced photoresponses. *J. Colloid. Interf. Sci.*, **353**:588–592.

[32] Chen ML, Liu JW, Hu B, Chen ML and Wang JH. (2011). Conjugation of quantum dots with graphene for fluorescence imaging of live cells. *Analyst.*, **136**:4277–4283.

[33] Jiang SD, Tang G, Ma YF, Hu Y and Song L. (2015). Synthesis of nitrogen-doped graphene-ZnS quantum dots composites with highly efficient visible light photodegradation. *Mater. Chem. Phys.*, **151**:34–42.

[34] Xue LP, Shen CF, Zheng MB, Lu HL, Li NW, Ji GB, Pan LJ and Cao JM. (2011). Hydrothermal synthesis of graphene-ZnS quantum dot nanocomposites. *Mater. Lett.*, **65**:198–200.

[35] Shi XF, Xia XY, Cui GW, Deng N, Zhao YQ, Zhuo LH and Tang B. (2015). Multiple exciton generation application of PbS quantum dots in ZnO@PbS/graphene oxide for enhanced photocatalytic activity. *Appl. Catal. B-Environ.*, **163**:123–128.

[36] Konstantatos G, Badioli M, Gaudreau L, Osmond J, Bernechea M, de Arquer FPG, de Arquer FPG, Gatti F and Koppens FHL. (2012). Hybrid graphene-quantum dot phototransistors with ultrahigh gain. *Nat. Nanotechnol.*, **7**:363–368.

[37] Sun L, Zhou XT, Zhang YG and Guo TL. (2015). Enhanced field emission of graphene-ZnO quantum dots hybrid structure. *J. Alloy Compd.*, **632**: 604–608.

[38] Hu HW, Ding JN, Qian JF, Li Y, Bai L and Yuan NY. (2014). Layered CoS/graphene nanocomposite as high catalytic counter electrodes for quantum dot-sensitized solar cells. *Mater. Lett.*, **114**:7–10.

[39] Zhou XY, Shi JJ, Liu Y, Su QM, Zhang J and Du GH. (2014). Microwave irradiation synthesis of Co3O4 quantum dots/graphene composite as anode materials for Li-ion battery. *Electrochim Acta.*, **143**:175–179.

[40] Yun DY, Park HM, Kim SW, Kim SW and Kim TW. (2014). Enhancement of memory margins for stable organic bistable devices based on graphene-oxide layers due to embedded CuInS2 quantum dots. *Carbon*, **75**:244–248.

Chapter 8

Magnetic Quantum Dot Hybrid Nanocomposites for Multimodal Cancer Imaging and Therapy

Semiconductor quantum dots (QDs) and magnetic materials both play very important roles in biomedicine. The development of nanocomposites that synchronously possess bright fluorescence and strong magnetism has attracted great attention because such materials can be used for bioseparation and multimodal cancer imaging and therapy. For instance, magnetic-fluorescent nanocomposites have been fabricated that can separate cancer cells and allow fluorescent identification, be used for both magnetic resonance and fluorescence imaging, and effectively kill cancer cells through synergistic photothermal and photodynamic effects. The methods of combining QDs and magnetic nanoparticles include seed-mediated growth, paramagnetic metal ion-doping, conjugating QDs onto magnetic nanoparticles using cross-linking agents and incorporating QDs and magnetic nanoparticles into spheres, etc. In this Chapter, the preparation methods and biomedical applications of QD-magnetic nanoparticle hybrid nanocomposites are discussed. The limitations of these nanocomposites are also considered.

1. Introduction

Magnetic nanoparticles composed of materials including iron (II,III) oxide (Fe_3O_4), maghemite (γ-Fe_2O_3), gadolinium chelates, iron and platinum

(FePt), cobalt and nickel, along with nonmagnetic nanocrystals doped with paramagnetic metal ions, have been fabricated. In the past decades, magnetic nanoparticles have attracted considerable attention globally because they have a variety of interesting biomedical applications, including magnetic resonance (MR) imaging, targeted drug delivery, bioseparation, and cancer therapy induced by near-infrared (NIR) laser or alternating magnetic field (AMF) [1–5]. Importantly, magnetic iron oxide nanoparticles exhibit no or ultralow toxicity and have been safely used clinically [6–9]. Magnetic iron oxide nanoparticles already have US Food Drug Administration (FDA) approval for clinical use [10].

When semiconductor QDs are combined with magnetic nanoparticles, the resulting nanocomposites may possess both fluorescence and magnetism, so they can be used for numerous interesting biofunctions, such as fluorescence and MR imaging, cell separation and identification, and photothermal therapy (PTT) and photodynamic therapy (PDT).

There are at least three methods used to combine QDs and magnetic nanoparticles. The first is direct growth of QDs on an iron-based magnetic nanostructure or doping QDs with paramagnetic metal ions. The second method involves incorporation of both QDs and magnetic nanoparticles into a nanocarrier like a polymer or silica (SiO_2) sphere. The third method is conjugation of QDs onto magnetic nanoparticles using cross-linking agents. The sizes of these novel magnetic-fluorescent hybrid composites (termed "magnetic QDs" in the following sections) made by different methods range from several nanometers to micrometers. Different methods are used to prepare magnetic QDs according to their intended applications. The development of magnetic QDs with low or no toxicity will promote the use of these magnetic fluorescent nanocomposites in clinical applications.

2. Synthesis of Magnetic QDs via Seed-mediated Growth or Doping with Paramagnetic Metal Ions

The magnetic-fluorescent nanocomposites synthesized via seed-mediated growth to date include FePt-cadmium sulfide (CdS) [11], FePt-cadmium selenide (CdSe) [12], FePt-zinc sulfide (ZnS) [13], γ-Fe_2O_3/CdS [14], γ-Fe_2O_3/ZnS [14], γ-Fe_2O_3/CdSe [15], Fe_3O_4/CdSe [16], Fe_3O_4/CdSe/ZnS

[15] and Fe_3O_4/CdSe quantum rods (QRs) [16], Ni-CdSe [17] and Fe_3O_4/$Cu_{2-X}S$ [18], etc. In 2004, Gu *et al.* [11] reported the direct chemical synthesis of heterodimers of nanoparticles with a size of around 7 nm that were composed of QDs and magnetic nanoparticles. The strategy used to form these asymmetrical dimers (heterodimers) of two different nanoparticles (CdS and FePt) is shown in Fig. 8.1a. This synthetic route involves four steps. First, FePt nanocrystals with a size of ~2.5 nm were synthesized in dioctyl ether in the presence of oleylamine and oleic acid. Second, sulfur powder was added to the unpurified FePt suspension at 100°C, where it was adsorbed by FePt to form an FePt/S (also written as FePt@S) core–shell nanocomposite. Third, cadmium acetylacetonate ($Cd(acac)_2$), trioctylphosphine oxide and hexadecane-1,2-diol were added to the

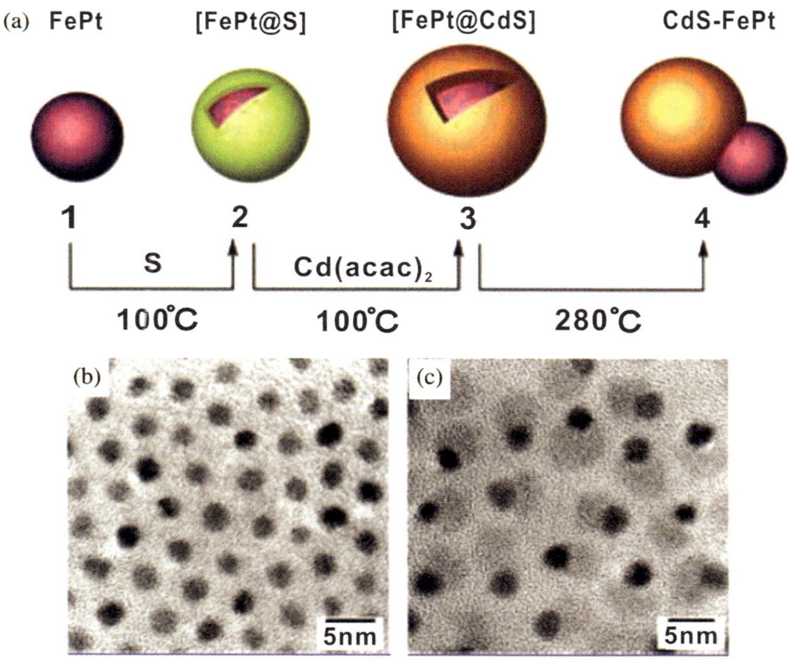

Fig. 8.1. Synthesis and morphology of an FePt/CdS nanocomposite. (a) Formation of the FePt/CdS nanocomposite. High-resolution transmission electron microscopy (TEM) images of (b) FePt and (c) FePt/CdS nanocomposite. Reprinted with permission from Ref. [11]. Copyright (2004) American Chemical Society.

FePt/S suspension. Fourth, the temperature of the mixture was increased from 100 to 280°C. The original FePt and final heterodimers of crystalline CdS and FePt nanoparticles are shown in Figs. 8.1b and 8.1c, respectively. CdS QDs grew directly on the surface of FePt, and the diameters of the FePt and CdS nanoparticles were 2.5 and ~3–4 nm, respectively. This synthetic process is simple, and the obtained FePt/CdS nanocomposites exhibited not only superparamagnetism, but also blue fluorescence with emission maxima at 438 nm. The fluorescent quantum yield of the FePt/CdS nanocomposite was about 3.2%.

However, CdS QDs are seldom used for bioimaging because their QY is low and CdS QDs that display red or NIR fluorescence are difficult to synthesize. Therefore, researchers selected other materials such as CdSe [15–17] and CdSe/ZnS [16] to prepare magnetic fluorescent nanocomposites. In 2011, Lin *et al.* [15] synthesized CdSe-decorated γ-Fe_2O_3 with multicolor emission and high QY by seed-mediated synthesis. Lin and colleagues first synthesized oleic acid-capped maghemite γ-Fe_2O_3 nanoparticles with a diameter of 8–10 nm. The main precursors including cadmium oxide (CdO), γ-Fe_2O_3 and selenium powder were then heated to 280–300°C for different time periods (Fig. 8.2a) to form γ-Fe_2O_3/CdSe nanocomposites with different morphologies. They hypothesized that heterodimers of γ-Fe_2O_3/CdSe would form when the growth time was short (1–2 min), as illustrated in Fig. 8.2b, left. However, for longer growth periods (e.g., 5–8 min), the γ-Fe_2O_3 cores were coated with three or more CdSe QDs (Fig. 8.2b, right). The saturation magnetization at 5 K of the superparamagnetic γ-Fe_2O_3/CdSe nanocomposites was 0.40 emu/g. The fluorescence of the nanocomposites could be tailored by controlling the growth of CdSe, and the QY of the nanocomposites ranged from 13% to 18%. To improve the solubility of the γ-Fe_2O_3/CdSe nanocomposites in water, they were coated with a SiO_2 shell. The resulting γ-Fe_2O_3/CdSe/SiO_2 core–shell nanocomposites with different fluorescence maxima retained high QYs of 8–13% (Fig. 8.2c). These magnetic fluorescent hybrid nanocomposites may have many potential biomedical applications.

QDs with different shapes, including QRs and core–shell QDs, can be grown on the surface of magnetic nanoparticles by seed-mediated synthesis. Recently, Cho *et al.* [16] used Fe_3O_4 nanoparticles as seeds for the

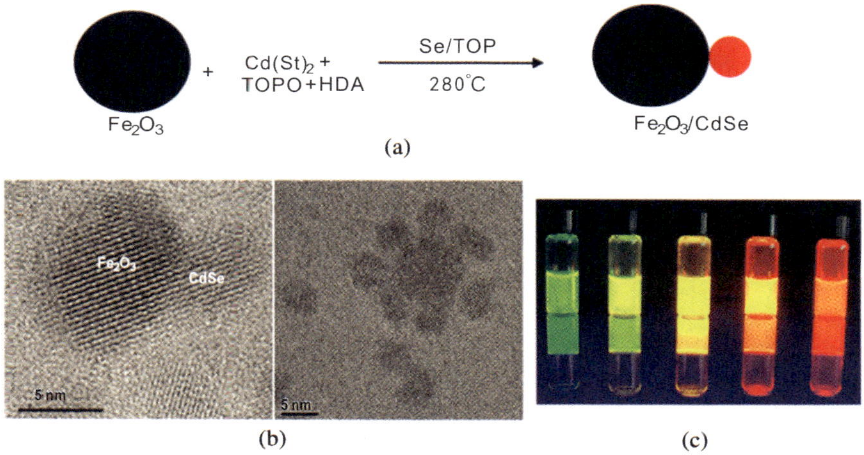

Fig. 8.2. Synthesis and properties of γ-Fe_2O_3/CdSe nanocomposites. (a) Formation of a γ-Fe_2O_3/CdSe heterodimer. (b) High-resolution TEM images of γ-Fe_2O_3/CdSe nanocomposites. Left: heterodimers; right: assembly of QDs around a γ-Fe_2O_3 nanoparticle. (c) True-color fluorescence of aqueous solutions of the SiO_2-coated γ-Fe_2O_3/CdSe nanocomposites. Reprinted with permission from Ref. [15]. Copyright (2011) Elsevier.

growth of CdSe QDs, CdSe QRs and CdSe/ZnS core–shell QDs. They used FeO(OH) and oleic acid as precursors to synthesize nearly monodisperse Fe_3O_4 nanocrystals through the pyrolysis of iron-oleate complexes at 320°C for 2 h under nitrogen flow. A solution of the Fe_3O_4 nanocrystals in hexanes was injected into a mixture of CdO, octadecylamine and 1-octadecene, which was then incubated at 280°C for 1 h under nitrogen flow. Selenium powder dissolved in trioctylphosphine was slowly added to the above mixture, which was subsequently reacted at 250°C for different periods to give Fe_3O_4 cores coated with CdSe QDs (Fig. 8.3a). Fe_3O_4 cores coated with CdSe QRs were synthesized using a similar method with different reaction and cooling temperatures and reaction times. Fe_3O_4/CdSe/ZnS nanocomposites were synthesized by mixing a solution of Fe_3O_4/CdSe with a mixture of ZnO and oleic acid in 1-octadecene at 220°C. All of the nanocomposites formed by this procedure possessed satisfactory optical and magnetic properties. For example, the Fe_3O_4/CdSe/ZnS QDs not only emitted bright fluorescence (QY: ~5%), but also could strongly attract to a magnet (Fig. 8.3b). The surface of each Fe_3O_4

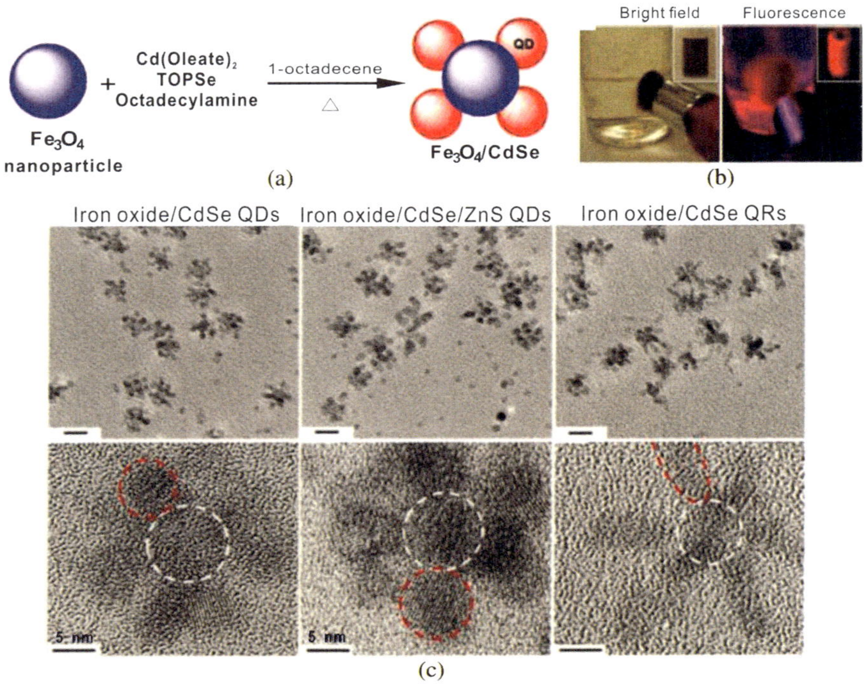

Fig. 8.3. Synthesis and properties of Fe_3O_4/CdSe nanocomposites with different morphologies. (a) Formation of a Fe_3O_4/CdSe nanocomposite. (b) Bright-field and fluorescence images of the Fe_3O_4/CdSe/ZnS complexes collected by a strong handheld magnet. Inset is the Fe_3O_4/CdSe/ZnS suspension without a magnetic field. (c) High-resolution TEM images of Fe_3O_4/CdSe QDs, Fe_3O_4/CdSe/ZnS QDs and Fe_3O_4/CdSe QRs. The white (in the center of the nanocomposites) and red dotted circles indicate Fe_3O_4 cores and QDs, respectively. Scale bars: 20 nm (upper) and 5 nm (lower). Reprinted with permission from Ref. [16]. Copyright (2014) American Chemical Society.

nanoparticle could provide several nucleation sites for QD growth. Therefore, each Fe_3O_4 nanoparticle was decorated with several QDs (or QRs), and the average width (length) of CdSe QDs, CdSe/ZnS QDs and CdSe QRs on the Fe_3O_4 nanoparticles were 3.5 ± 0.4 (4.4 ± 0.6), 4.9 ± 0.6 (6.7 ± 0.9), and 3.7 ± 0.4 (7.8 ± 0.8) nm, respectively, as shown in Fig. 8.3c.

It is known that cadmium (Cd) is toxic to cells and animals and a probable carcinogen. Therefore, magnetic-fluorescent nanocomposites with Cd-free QDs may be more useful than those with Cd-containing QDs. Copper (Cu)-containing QDs exhibit lower toxicity than Cd-containing ones. In 2013, Tian *et al.* [18] synthesized $Fe_3O_4/Cu_{2-x}S$ core–shell nanocomposites (Fig. 8.4a). In their experiments, sulfur dissolved in oleylamine was added to a solution of Fe_3O_4 nanoparticles in

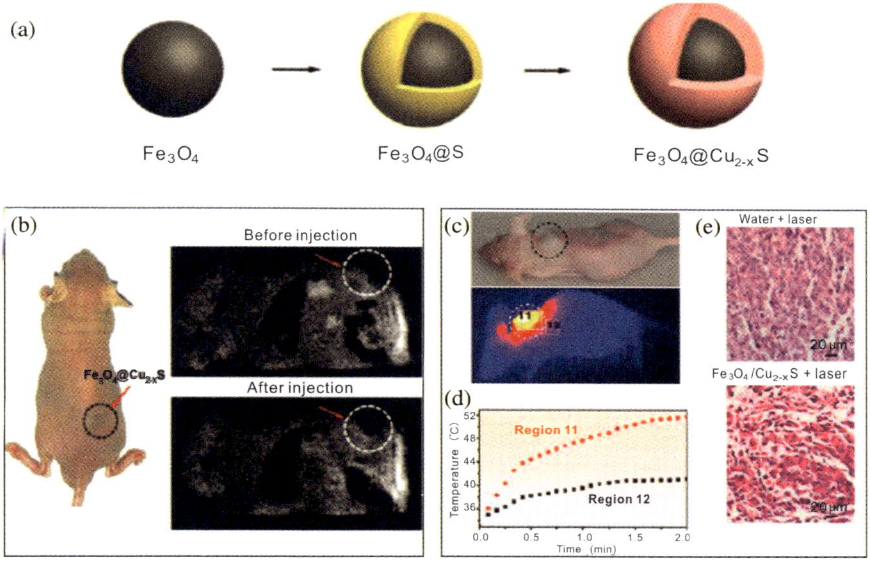

Fig. 8.4. (a) Schematic illustration of the formation of an $Fe_3O_4/Cu_{2-x}S$ core–shell nanocomposite. (b) Use of the polymer-coated $Fe_3O_4/Cu_{2-x}S$ nanocomposite for *in vivo* MR imaging. (c) Use of the polymer-coated $Fe_3O_4/Cu_{2-x}S$ nanocomposite for *in vivo* infrared thermal imaging. The tumor containing the $Fe_3O_4/Cu_{2-x}S$ nanocomposite was irradiated with a 980 nm laser for 2 min. The injection site is indicated by a dashed circle. (d) The temperature of the tumor and a surrounding site increased with irradiation time. This mouse is the same as that shown in (c). (e) Use of the polymer-coated $Fe_3O_4/Cu_{2-x}S$ nanocomposite for *in vivo* cancer PTT. These are hematoxylin and eosin-stained histological images. Upper: tumor + water + 980 nm laser, lower: tumor + $Fe_3O_4/Cu_{2-x}S$ nanocomposite + 980 nm laser (cell shrinkage, loss of contact, and nuclear damage were observed in this image). Reprinted with permission from Ref. [18]. Copyright (2013) American Chemical Society.

cyclohexane at 70°C. Copper acetylacetonate ($Cu(acac)_2$) dissolved in chloroform and oleylamine was then injected into the Fe_3O_4-S suspension, which was reacted at 70°C. A thin $Cu_{2-x}S$ shell grew on the surface of the Fe_3O_4 nanoparticles. The as-prepared $Fe_3O_4/Cu_{2-x}S$ nanocomposites were then coated with an amphiphilic hydrolyzed polymaleic anhydride pre-modified with oleylamine. The obtained polymer-coated $Fe_3O_4/Cu_{2-x}S$ core–shell nanocomposites show ability for T2-weighted MR imaging and infrared thermal imaging as well as cancer PTT. As shown in Fig. 8.4b, when the polymer-coated $Fe_3O_4/Cu_{2-x}S$ nanocomposite (100 μL, 20 ppm Fe) was injected into the back of a mouse (~0.2 cm deep, dosage: 0.14 mg/kg), T2-weighted MR imaging showed that the gray degree at the injection site obviously decreased after injection. After a tumor-bearing mouse was intratumorally injected with the polymer-coated $Fe_3O_4/Cu_{2-x}S$ nanocomposite (100 μL, 50 ppm Cu) and irradiated with a 980 nm laser (0.6 W/cm^2), the *in vivo* infrared thermal image captured by a PTT monitoring system showed that the thermal signal at the tumor site was much higher than that of the surrounding tissue, and the temperature at the tumor site increased with irradiation time (Figs. 8.4c and 8.4d). In addition, the tumor tissue treated with the polymer-coated $Fe_3O_4/Cu_{2-x}S$ nanocomposite and NIR laser irradiation showed obvious damage compared with tumor tissue in the control mouse (Fig. 8.4e).

In the magnetic-fluorescent nanocomposites described above, QDs grow directly on the surface of the magnetic particles. The fluorescent QY of this kind of nanocomposite is usually low because energy can be easily transferred from the QD shell to the magnetic core. To overcome this limitation, Ding and colleagues [19] doped the ZnS shells of copper indium sulfide ($CuInS_2$) QDs with manganese (Mn) to form a $CuInS_2$/ZnS:Mn nanocomposite. First, they coated $CuInS_2$ seed crystals with a ZnS shell at 230°C using zinc stearate as a precursor. Mn stearate was added to the unpurified $CuInS_2$/ZnS solution, which was then heated at 180°C. The diameter of the as-prepared $CuInS_2$/ZnS:Mn nanocomposite particles was only 3.6 ± 0.6 nm. These Mn-doped QDs exhibited bright red fluorescence (emission range: ~550–750 nm) and their QY exceeded 27%. To improve their solubility in water, the $CuInS_2$/ZnS:Mn nanocomposite was modified with dihydrolipoic acid–polyethylene glycol (DHLA–PEG). The PEGylated $CuInS_2$/ZnS:Mn QDs (0.4 μmoL QDs) were intravenously injected into mice with tumors grown from S180 cells. *In vivo* fluorescence imaging revealed that the maximum fluorescence signal was observed in the tumor about 6 h post-injection (Fig. 8.5a). The whole accumulation and loss process of the $CuInS_2$/ZnS:Mn QDs in the tumor was observed in real time through *in vivo* fluorescence imaging. These $CuInS_2$/ZnS:Mn QDs were also used for tumor MR imaging. After tumor-bearing mice were intratumorally injected with the PEGylated $CuInS_2$/ ZnS:Mn QDs, the T1 value of the tumor region started to decrease and

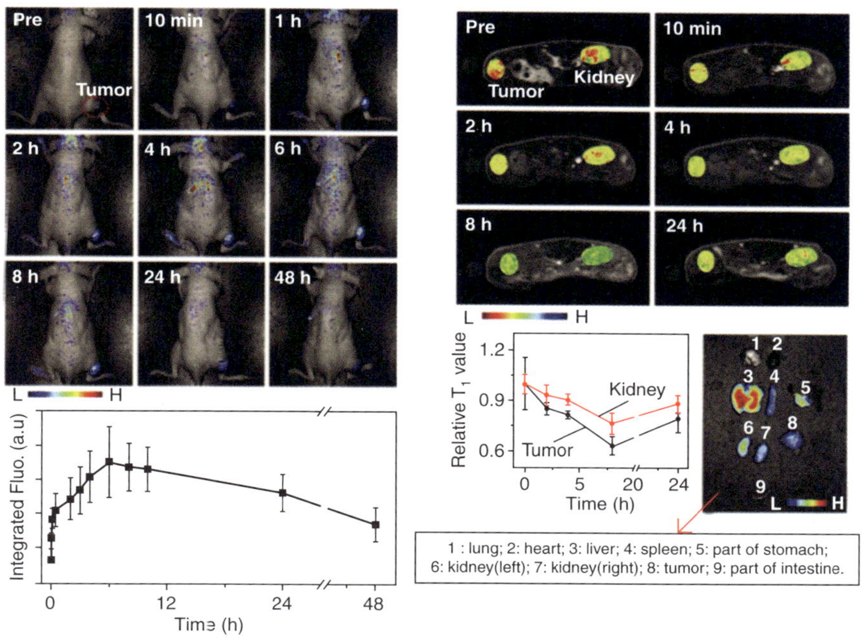

(a) (b)

Fig. 8.5. PEGylated $CuInS_2$/ZnS:Mn QDs injected into the tail vein of tumor-bearing mice for fluorescent and MR imaging. (a) Upper frame: PEGylated $CuInS_2$/ZnS:Mn QDs targeting the mouse tumor (indicated by the red dashed circle) monitored by *in vivo* fluorescence imaging. Lower frame: temporal evolution of the integrated fluorescence signals recorded from the tumor region. (b) Upper frame: MR imaging (T1-weighted MR images); right frame of the lower panel: *ex vivo* fluorescence images of main organs harvested 24 h post-injection; left frame of the lower panel: temporal T1 values of tumor and kidney sites. Reprinted with permission from Ref. [19]. Copyright (2014) Elsevier.

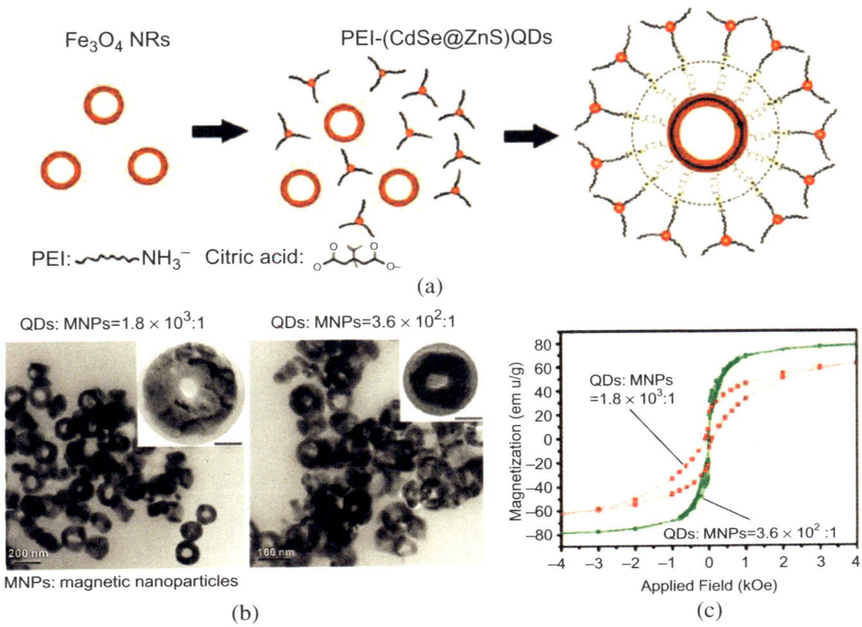

Fig. 8.6. Preparation and properties of QD-capped magnetite nanorings. (a) Schematic illustrations of the formation of nanocomposites by mixing PEI-capped CdSe/ZnS and citric acid-capped magnetite nanorings (NRs). (b) TEM images and (c) hysteresis loops of the nanocomposites prepared from different ratios of QDs to magnetic nanoparticles. Reprinted with permission from Ref. [21]. Copyright (2010) American Chemical Society.

reached a minimum 8 h after injection (Fig. 8.5b). Therefore, these $CuInS_2$/ZnS:Mn QDs are dual-modality imaging probes that may have potential for cancer diagnosis.

3. Formation of Magnetic QDs by Conjugating QDs onto Magnetic Nanoparticles through Cross-linking Agents

To limit fluorescence quenching of QDs by magnetic nanoparticles, QDs can be conjugated onto magnetic nanoparticles through cross-linking agents [20–28]. The cross-linkers may prevent or reduce the transfer of charge from QDs to magnetic nanoparticles when the nanocomposites are excited by an external light. Although QDs can grow on the cross-linkers in most of the methods used to prepare such magnetic-fluorescent nanosystems, both QDs and magnetic nanoparticles are synthesized before combination. This allows researchers to construct the nanocomposites from high-quality QDs and magnetic nanoparticles.

In 2011, Kale *et al.* [20] reported a strategy to prepare bifunctional nanocomposites composed of Fe_3O_4 nanoparticles and cadmium telluride (CdTe) QDs using dodecylamine (DDA) as a cross linker. To fabricate the CdTe-decorated magnetic nanoparticles, they synthesized citric acid-coated Fe_3O_4 nanoparticles, which were then coated with DDA through covalent reaction. The resulting Fe_3O_4/DDA nanoparticles were used as a nucleation matrix for CdTe QDs by adsorbing Cd^{2+} ions and mercaptopropionic acid. After the addition of sodium hydrogen telluride, CdTe nanocrystals formed on the Fe_3O_4/DDA nanoparticles at pH 9 and 100°C. In the as-prepared Fe_3O_4/DDA/CdTe nanocomposites, CdTe were separately deposited on the magnetic nanoparticle surface, but were not in core–shell form. The Fe_3O_4/DDA/CdTe nanocomposites exhibited strong saturation magnetization (44 emu/g) and fluorescence (QY: 18 ± 2%). As a result, when these magnetic fluorescent nanocomposites were conjugated with anti-epidermal growth factor receptor (EGFR) antibody, the bioconjugates could be used to efficiently separate and image the EGFR-positive leukemic Molt-4 cells from a mixed suspension of cells of the same size.

QDs can be assembled on the surface of magnetic nanoparticles; e.g., by electrostatic interaction between the QDs and linkers on the nanoparticle surface. In 2010, Fan and co-workers [21] constructed magnetic fluorescent nanocomposites by mixing cationic polyethylenimine (PEI)-capped CdSe/ZnS QDs with negatively charged magnetite nanorings modified with citric acid (Fig. 8.6a). QDs were strongly bound to the magnetite nanorings through electrostatic attraction. The diameter and fluorescence properties of the as-prepared nanocomposites could be conveniently tailored by changing the ratio of QDs to magnetic nanoparticles and the size or type of QDs. The magnetism of the nanocomposites was also influenced by the amount of QDs on the surface of the magnetic nanoparticles. As shown in Fig. 8.6b, when the ratio of CdSe/ZnS QDs to magnetic nanoparticles was increased from 360:1 to 1800:1, the average diameter of the resulting nanocomposites increased from 100 ± 10 to 210 ± 20 nm, and their saturation magnetization obviously decreased.

Xu *et al*. [22] prepared a multifunctional nanocomposite with Fe_3O_4 cores and CdSe/ZnS QDs by this assembly method. They coated Fe_3O_4 nanoparticles with a SiO_2 shell that was then modified with thiol (–SH) groups. the resulting Fe_3O_4/SiO_2-SH core–shell nanoparticles were mixed with mercaptopropionic acid (MPA)-capped CdSe/ZnS QDs, causing the MPA-QDs to deposit on the Fe_3O_4/SiO_2-SH nanoparticles by thiol coordination (Fig. 8.7a). Although the magnetism of the Fe_3O_4/SiO_2-CdSe/ZnS

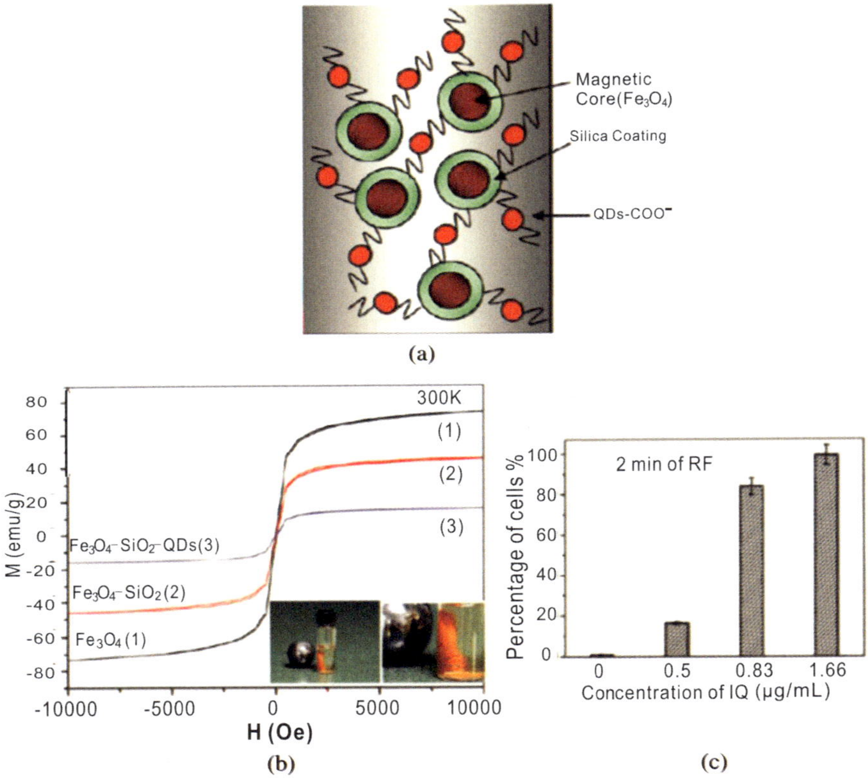

Fig. 8.7. Fe_3O_4/SiO_2-CdSe/ZnS nanocomposites prepared by an assembly method for cancer treatment. (a) Schematic illustrations of CdSe/ZnS QD-decorated Fe_3O_4/SiO_2 nanocomposites. (b) Hysteresis curves of the samples. Inset: Separation of a Fe_3O_4/SiO_2–CdSe/ZnS nanocomposite in solution using a magnetic ball (left: low magnification; right: high magnification). (c) The ability of the Fe_3O_4/SiO_2-CdSe/ZnS to kill human pancreatic cancer cells upon 2 min of RF treatment. Reprinted with permission from Ref. [22]. Copyright (2010) American Chemical Society.

nanocomposite was lower than that of Fe_3O_4 and Fe_3O_4/SiO_2 nanoparticles, the material still had a high saturation magnetization (15.4 emu/g), as indicated in Fig. 8.7b. When human pancreatic cancer cells (Panc-1) were incubated with the Fe_3O_4/SiO_2-CdSe/ZnS nanocomposite and then irradiated by a radio frequency (RF) of 350 kHz (5 kW), the cells were killed in a short time (2 min), and the death rate of the cells increased with nanocomposite concentration (Fig. 8.7c). Cell death was induced by the nanocomposites generating heat during RF exposure. Meanwhile, almost all of the cells that were incubated with nanocomposites without RF treatment and RF alone as control experiments survived. Because this low-frequency radiation can penetrate biological tissues, the use of magnetic QD nanocomposites in RF treatment has potential for cancer therapy.

Besides RF, NIR light also has the ability to induce Fe_3O_4 and semiconductor QDs to kill cancer cells. Upon laser irradiation, both Fe_3O_4 and semiconductor QDs can efficiently convert NIR laser light into heat in a short time [5, 23]. In addition, QDs can generate reactive oxygen species (ROS) upon laser irradiation [23]. Therefore, the magnetic-fluorescent nanocomposites described above can be used not only for bioimaging and bioseparation, but also for cancer PTT and PDT.

4. Formation of Magnetic QDs by Incorporating QDs and Magnetic Nanoparticles into Spheres

The magnetic-fluorescent nanocomposites constructed by growing QDs directly on magnetic nanoparticles or by conjugation through cross-linking agents are difficult to load with a large amount of drugs, which may limit their use in multimodal cancer treatment. Therefore, it is necessary to develop nanosystems that can synchronously load QDs, magnetic nanoparticles and drugs. Polymers and SiO_2 are usually used as carriers to fabricate magnetic-fluorescent nanocomposites [29–35]. For example, magnetic polystyrene nanospheres (MPNs) have been used for loading CdTe QDs [29]. The saturation magnetization and QY of the resulting novel polymer nanospheres (MPN/CdTe) were 15.7 emu/g and 2%, respectively. After conjugation of epidermal growth factor (EGF), the nanobioconjugates could not only label cancer cells that over-expressed EGFR, but could also rapidly separate these cancer cells. Antibody-conjugated magnetic–fluorescent nanospheres for labeling and separation of cancer cells also have been developed [30]. As shown in Fig. 8.8a, MPNs were coated with CdTe/CdS core–shell QDs through electrostatic adsorption, and the MPN-QD composite obtained was then coated with a SiO_2 shell (denoted MPN-QDs-SiO_2). Anti-EGFR antibodies (12H23) were then conjugated onto the nanocomposite. Scanning electron microscopy (SEM) images showed that the average diameters of the MPN, MPN–QDs and MPN-QDs-SiO_2 samples were 746.12 ±

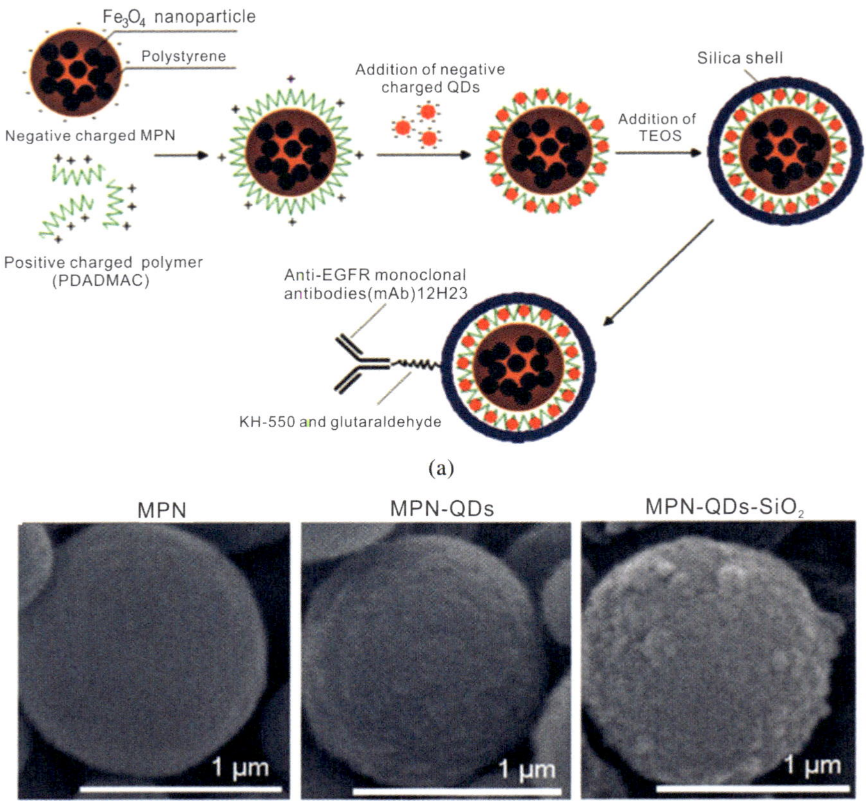

(a)

(b)

Fig. 8.8. Preparation and morphology of magnetic–fluorescent polymer nanospheres. (a) Schematic illustration of the formation of antibody-conjugated MPN-QDs-SiO_2. (b) SEM images of MPN, MPN-QDs, and MPN-QDs-SiO_2. Reprinted with permission from Ref. [30]. Copyright (2010) Springer.

583.34, 791.81 ± 510.20, and 813.61 ± 602.00 nm, respectively (Fig. 8.8b). The MPN–QDs–SiO_2 composite may exhibit low toxicity compared with the uncoated MPN–QDs one because of the presence of the SiO_2 shell. The 12H23-conjugated MPN-QDs-SiO_2 bioconjugate readily recognized breast cancer cells (e.g., MDA-MB-435S), which was easily confirmed by fluorescence imaging. Furthermore, these bioconjugates could specifically and quickly separate cancer cells via magnetic force.

Although Fe_3O_4 nanoparticles have strong continuous absorption spectra that cover the visible and NIR regions, QD fluorescence is not easily quenched by the Fe_3O_4 nanoparticles in the two kinds of magnetic-fluorescent nanospheres described above [29, 30]. This is because the Fe_3O_4 nanoparticles were coated with thick polymer (polystyrene) shell, and the QDs were adsorbed onto this shell rather than directly onto the magnetic nanoparticles. However, if QDs and Fe_3O_4 nanoparticles are synchronously encapsulated into a polymer matrix, the QY of the QDs may decrease considerably because the QDs may directly contact the surface of the Fe_3O_4 nanoparticles, which facilitates energy transfer. To overcome this limitation, Tu *et al.* [31] coated Fe_3O_4 nanoparticles with a SiO_2 shell and CdTe QDs with didecyl-p-vinylbenzylmethylammonium chloride (DVMAC), and then simultaneously encapsulated both Fe_3O_4/SiO_2 and CdTe/DVMAC into polystyrene microspheres. The resulting bifunctional polystyrene microspheres exhibited both bright fluorescence and strong magnetism.

Polystyrene is not suitable for *in vivo* applications because it is not easily degraded in the body. In 2014, Ye *et al.* [32] used poly(lactic-co-glycolic acid) (PLGA) to encapsulate Fe_3O_4 nanoparticles, manganese-doped zinc sulfide (Mn:ZnS) QDs and anticancer drug busulfan, as shown in Fig. 8.9a. PLGA is a biodegradable polymer that has been approved by the FDA for therapeutic applications. The resulting PLGA-Fe_3O_4-Mn:ZnS nanocomposite had an average diameter of about 93 nm, making them suitable for intravenous injection. The PLGA-Fe_3O_4-Mn:ZnS nanocomposite exhibited bright fluorescence (emission peak: 599 nm) and superparamagnetism. When murine J774A macrophage cells were incubated with the PLGA-Fe_3O_4-Mn:ZnS nanocomposite, the migration of the nanocomposite particles into cells could be observed via fluorescence imaging. The cells continuously took up the PLGA-Fe_3O_4-Mn:ZnS nanocomposite

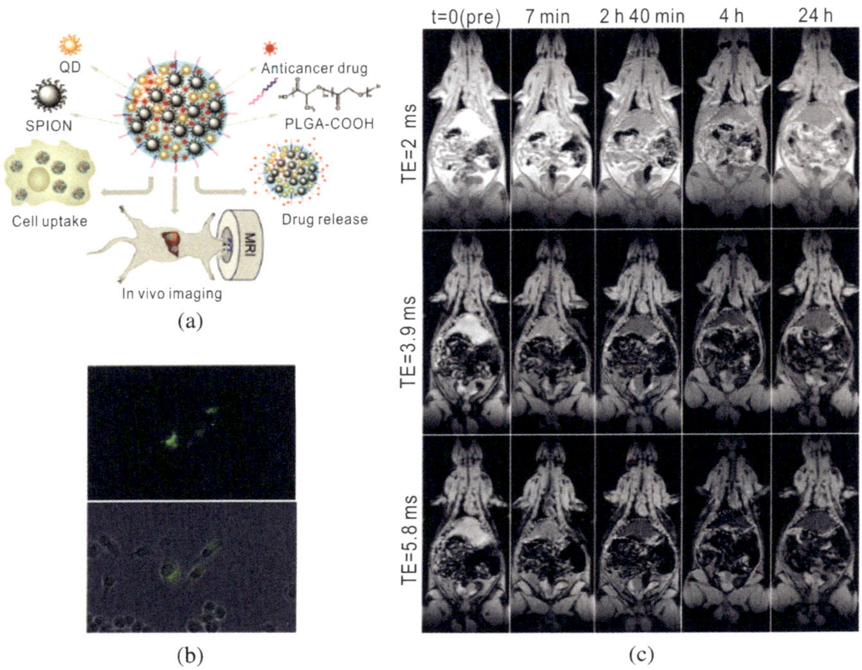

Fig. 8.9. PLGA-Fe_3O_4-Mn:ZnS nanocomposite for fluorescence and MR imaging. (a) Schematic illustration of the formation of the PLGA-Fe_3O_4-Mn:ZnS nanocomposite and its multiple applications. (b) Fluorescence and fluorescence-bright field merged images of murine J774A macrophage cells incubated with the nanocomposite for 24 h. (c) T2-weighted *in vivo* MR images of a rat before and after intravenous injection of the nanocomposite. The liver is encircled by white dashed lines. Reprinted with permission from Ref. [32]. Copyright (2010) Elsevier.

and emitted the brightest fluorescence after incubation for 24 h, which was conveniently confirmed by fluorescence imaging (Fig. 8.9b). When the PLGA-Fe_3O_4-Mn:ZnS nanocomposite was intravenously injected into rats with a weight of 500 g, T2-weighted MR images showed that the signals from the liver and spleen rapidly decreased after injection (Fig. 8.9c). Especially in the MR images taken with longer echo times (e.g., 5.8 ms), the signal from the liver was close to black 24 h post-injection. MR imaging also revealed that a small amount of the nanocomposite migrated into the kidneys, but almost none was observed in the brain and testes. The as-prepared PLGA–Fe_3O_4–Mn:ZnS nanocomposite also showed high entrapment efficiency (89 ± 2%) for the lipophilic drug busulfan and sustained drug release over a period of 5 weeks.

5. Discussion

Magnetic nanoparticles and semiconductor QDs respectively exhibit excellent magnetic and optical properties. Hybrid nanocomposites composed of magnetic nanoparticles and semiconductor QDs can be used for not only cancer fluorescence and MR imaging, but also cancer PTT and PDT induced by red or NIR laser irradiation, as well as hyperthermia cancer therapy induced by an AMF. Magnetic–fluorescent hybrid nanocomposites may also have other novel functions. For example, magnetic nanoparticles can destroy cancer cells through magnetomechanical force under a low-frequency AMF [36–40]. Therefore, hybrid nanocomposites may also vibrate, oscillate, or rotate under a magnetic field and then transfer mechanical force to cancer cells. Apoptosis of cancer cells could be induced by magnetic switching by controlling cancer cell death signaling [41, 42]. If magnetic-fluorescent hybrid nanocomposites are conjugated with anti-death receptor monoclonal antibody and then incubated with cancer cells, cell apoptosis should occur through aggregation of the death receptors after the cells are exposed to a magnetic field. Overall, magnetic-fluorescent hybrid nanocomposites possess numerous functions for cancer therapy.

It should be noted that when these two different kinds of nanomaterials are directly combined with each other or incorporated into a matrix together, the saturation magnetization and fluorescent QY of the hybrid nanocomposites usually decrease substantially compared with the corresponding properties of the magnetic nanoparticles and QDs alone. The saturation magnetization and fluorescence of hybrid nanocomposites also tend to decrease during storage. Magnetic nanoparticles not only quench QD fluorescence, but also lower the level of intracellular ROS generated by the QDs. Therefore, the efficacy of PDT using hybrid nanocomposites may be considerably lower than that of QDs alone. In addition, hybrid nanocomposites tend to be much larger than magnetic nanoparticles and QDs alone, which also limits their ability in *in vivo* targeted imaging and therapy. Magnetic iron oxide nanoparticles have FDA approval for clinical use, but QDs, especially Cd-containing ones, are usually highly toxic to cells and animals. Therefore, the hybrid nanocomposites developed to date may not be suitable for use in vivo in humans because of their toxicity.

References

[1] Zhang L, Xue H, Gao CL, Carr L, Wang JN, Chu BC and Jiang SY. (2010). Imaging and cell targeting characteristics of magnetic nanoparticles modified by a functionalizable zwitterionic polymer with adhesive 3,4-dihydroxyphenyl-L-alanine linkages. *Biomaterials*, **31**:6582–6588.

[2] Lee JH, Jang JT, Choi JS, Moon SH, Noh SH, Kim JW, Kim JG, Kim IS, Park KI and Cheon J. (2011). Exchange-coupled magnetic nanoparticles for efficient heat induction. *Nat. Nanotechnol.*, **6**:418–422.

[3] Laurent S and Mahmoudi M. (2011). Superparamagnetic iron oxide nanoparticles: promises for diagnosis and treatment of cancer. *Int. J. Mol. Epidemiol. Genet.*, **2**:24.

[4] Yang HW, Hua MY, Liu HL, Huang CY, Tsai RY, Lu YJ, Chen JY, Hsien HY, Chang YS, Yen TC, Chen PY and Wei KC. (2011). Self-protecting core-shell magnetic nanoparticles for targeted, traceable, long half-life delivery of BCNU to gliomas. *Biomaterials*, **32**:6523–6532.

[5] Chu MQ, Shao YX, Peng JL, Dai XY, Li HK, Wu QS, and Shi D. (2013). Near-infrared laser light mediated cancer therapy by photothermal effect of Fe_3O_4 magnetic nanoparticles. *Biomaterials*, **34**:4078–4088.

[6] Maier-Hauff K, Ulrich F, Nestler D, Niehoff H, Wust P, Thiesen B, Orawa H, Budach V and Jordan A. (2011). Efficacy and safety of intratumoral thermotherapy using magnetic iron-oxide nanoparticles combined with external beam radiotherapy on patients with recurrent glioblastoma multiforme. *J. Neuro-Oncol.*, **103**:317–324.

[7] Maier-Hauff K, Rothe R, Scholz R, Gneveckow U, Wust P, Thiesen B, Feusser A, von Deimling A, Waldoefner N, Felix R and Jordon A. (2007). Intracranial thermotherapy using magnetic nanoparticles combined with external beam radiotherapy: Results of a feasibility study on patients with glioblastoma multiforme. *J. Neuro-Oncol.*, **81**:53–60.

[8] Johannsen M, Gneueckow U, Thiesen B, Taymoorian K, Cho CH, Waldofner N, Scholz R, Jordan A, Loening SA and Wust P. (2007). Thermotherapy of prostate cancer using magnetic nanoparticles: feasibility, imaging, and three-dimensional temperature distribution. *Eur. Urol.*, **52**:1653–1662.

[9] Johannsen M, Gneveckow U, Taymoorian K, Thiesen B, Waldofner N, Scholz R, Jung K, Jordon A, Wust P and Loening SA. (2007). Morbidity and quality of life during thermotherapy using magnetic nanoparticles in locally recurrent prostate cancer: results of a prospective phase I trial. *Int. J. Hyperther.*, **23**:315–323.

[10] Jordan A, Scholz R, Maier-Hauff K, Johannsen M, Wust P, Nadobny J, Schirra H, Schmidt H, Deger S, Loening S, Lanksch W and Felix R. (2001). Presentation of a new magnetic field therapy system for the treatment of human solid tumors with magnetic fluid hyperthermia. *J. Magn. Magn. Mater.*, **225**:118–126.

[11] Gu HW, Zheng RK, Zhang XX and Xu B. (2004). Facile one-pot synthesis of bifunctional heterodimers of nanoparticles: a conjugate of quantum dot and magnetic nanoparticles. *J. Am. Chem. Soc.*, **126**:5664–5665.

[12] Gao JH, Zhang B, Gao Y, Pan Y, Zhang XX and Xu B. (2007). Fluorescent magnetic nanocrystals by sequential addition of reagents in a one-pot reaction: a simple preparation for multifunctional nanostructures. *J. Am. Chem. Soc.*, **129**:11928–11935.

[13] Gu HW, Zheng RK, Liu H, Zhang XX and Xu B. (2005). Direct synthesis of a bimodal nanosponge based on FePt and ZnS. *Small*, **1**:402–406.

[14] Kwon KW and Shim M. (2005). Gamma-Fe2O3/II-VI sulfide nanocrystal heterojunctions. *J. Am. Chem. Soc.*, **127**:10269–10275.

[15] Lin AWH, Ang CY, Patra PK, Han Y, Gu H, Le Breton JM, Juraszek J, Chiron H, Papaefthymiou GC, Selvan ST and Ying JY. (2011). Seed-mediated synthesis, properties and application of gamma-Fe2O3-CdSe magnetic quantum dots. *J Solid State Chem.*, **184**:2150–2158.

[16] Cho M, Contreras EQ, Lee SS, Jones CJ, Jang W and Colvin VL. (2014). Characterization and optimization of the fluorescence of nanoscale iron oxide/quantum dot complexes. *J. Phys. Chem. C.*, **118**:14606–14616.

[17] Siah WR, LaGrow AP, Banholzer MJ and Tilley RD. (2013). CdSe quantum dot growth on magnetic nickel nanoparticles. *Cryst. Growth Des.*, **13**:2486–2492.

[18] Tian Q, Hu J, Zhu Y, Zou R, Chen Z, Yang S, Li R, Su Q, Han Y and Liu X. (2013). Sub-10 nm $Fe_3O_4@Cu_{2-x}S$ Core–Shell Nanoparticles for Dual-Modal Imaging and Photothermal Therapy. *J. Am. Chem. Soc.*, **135**:8571–8577.

[19] Ding K, Jing LH, Liu CY, Hou Y and Gao MY. (2014). Magnetically engineered Cd-free quantum dots as dual-modality probes for fluorescence/magnetic resonance imaging of tumors. *Biomaterials*, **35**:1608–1617.

[20] Kale A, Kale S, Yadav P, Gholap H, Pasricha R, Jog JP, Lefez B, Hannoyer B, Shastry P and Ogale S. (2011). Magnetite/CdTe magnetic-fluorescent composite nanosystem for magnetic separation and bio-imaging. *Nanotechnology*. **22**:225101

[21] Fan HM, Olivo M, Shuter B, Yi JB, Bhuvaneswari R, Tan HR, Xing GC, NQ CT, Liu L, Lucky SS, Bay BH and Ding J. (2010). Quantum dot capped magnetite nanorings as high performance nanoprobe for multiphoton fluorescence and magnetic resonance imaging. *J. Am. Chem Soc.*, **132**:14803–14811.

[22] Xu Y, Karmakar A, Wang DY, Mahmood MW, Watanabe F, Zhang YB, Fejleh A, Fejleh P, Li Z, Kannarpady G, Ali S, Biris AR and Biris AS. (2010). Multifunctional Fe3O4 cored magnetic-quantum dot fluorescent nanocomposites for RF nanohyperthermia of cancer cells. *J. Phys. Chem. C.*, **114**:5020–5026.

[23] Chu MQ, Pan XJ, Zhang D, Wu Q, Peng JL and Hai WX. (2012). The therapeutic efficacy of CdTe and CdSe quantum dots for photothermal cancer therapy. *Biomaterials*, **33**:7071–7083.

[24] Yang HS, Santra S, Walter GA and Holloway PH. (2006). Gd-III-functionalized fluorescent quantum dots as multimodal imaging probes. *Adv. Mater.*, **18**:2890.

[25] Fernandez B, Galvez N, Cuesta R, Hungria AB, Calvino JJ and Dominguez-Vera JM. (2008). Quantum dots decorated with magnetic bionanoparticles. *Adv. Funct. Mater.*, **18**:3931–3935.

[26] Thakur D, Deng S, Baldet T and Winter JO. (2009). pH sensitive CdS-iron oxide fluorescent-magnetic nanocomposites. *Nanotechnology*, **20**:485601.

[27] Li LL, Li HB, Chen D, Liu HY, Tang FQ, Zhang YQ, Ren J and Li Y. (2009). Preparation and Characterization of Quantum Dots Coated Magnetic Hollow Spheres for Magnetic Fluorescent Multimodal Imaging and Drug Delivery. *J. Nanosci. Nanotechno*, **9**:2540–2545.

[28] Koktysh D, Bright V and Pham W. (2011). Fluorescent magnetic hybrid nanoprobe for multimodal bioimaging. *Nanotechnology*, **22**(27):275606.

[29] Chu MQ, Song X, Cheng D, Liu SP and Zhu J. (2006). Preparation of quantum dot-coated magnetic polystyrene nanospheres for cancer cell labelling and separation. *Nanotechnology*, **17**:3268–3273.

[30] Wu YC, Chu MQ, Shi BZ and Li ZH. (2011). A novel magneto-fluorescent nano-bioprobe for cancer cell targeting, imaging and collection. *Appl. Biochem. Biotech.*, **163**:813–825.

[31] Tu CF, Yang YH and Gao MY. (2008). Preparations of bifunctional polymeric beads simultaneously incorporated with fluorescent quantum dots and magnetic nanocrystals. *Nanotechnology*, **19**(10):105601.

[32] Ye F, Barrefelt A, Asem H, Abedi-Valugerdi M, El-Serafi I, Saghafian M, Abu-Salah K, Alrokayan S, Muhammed M and Hassan M. (2014). Biodegradable polymeric vesicles containing magnetic nanoparticles, quantum dots and anticancer drugs for drug delivery and imaging. *Biomaterials*, **35**:3885–3894.

[33] Zebli B, Susha AS, Sukhorukov GB, Rogach AL and Parak WJ. (2005). Magnetic targeting and cellular uptake of polymer microcapsules simultaneously functionalized with magnetic and luminescent nanocrystals. *Langmuir*, **21**:4262–4265.

[34] Sathe TR, Agrawal A and Nie SM. (2006). Mesoporous silica beads embedded with semiconductor quantum dots and iron oxide nanocrystals: Dual-function microcarriers for optical encoding and magnetic separation. *Anal. Chem.*, **78**:5627–5632.

[35] Xie YS, Wu YC, Chu MQ, Yu XY and Wu QS. (2013). A highly efficient route for preparing porous magnetic nanospheres with surface-adsorbed quantum dots. *J. Exp. Nanosci.*, **8**:588–597.

[36] Kim DH, Rozhkova EA, Ulasov IV, Bader SD, Rajh T, Lesniak MS and Novosad V. (2010). Biofunctionalized Magnetic-Vortex Microdiscs for Targeted Cancer-Cell Destruction. *Nat. Mater.*, **9**: 165–171.

[37] Domenech M, Marrero-Berrios I, Torres-Lugo M and Rinaldi C. (2013). Lysosomal membrane permeabilization by targeted magnetic nanoparticles in alternating magnetic fields. *ACS nano.*, **7**:5091–5101.

[38] Zhang EM, Kircher MF, Koch M, Eliasson L, Goldberg SN and Renstrom E. (2014). Dynamic magnetic fields remote-control apoptosis via nanoparticle rotation. *ACS Nano.*, **8**:3192–3201.

[39] Cheng DF, Li X, Zhang GX and Shi HC. (2014). Morphological Effect of oscillating magnetic nanoparticles in killing tumor cells. *Nanoscale Res. Lett.*, **9**:195.

[40] Wo FJ, Xu RJ, Shao YX, Zhang ZY, Chu MQ, Shi DL, Liu SP. (2016). A Multimodal System with Synergistic Effects of Magneto-Mechanical, Photothermal, Photodynamic and Chemo Therapies of Cancer in Graphene-Quantum Dot-Coated Hollow Magnetic Nanospheres. *Theranostics* **6**: 485–500.

[41] Mannix RJ, Kumar S, Cassiola F, Montoya-Zavala M, Feinstein E, Prentiss M and Ingber DE. (2008). Nanomagnetic actuation of receptor-mediated signal transduction. *Nature Nanotechnol.*, **3**:36–40.

[42] Cho MH, Lee EJ, Son M, Lee JH, Yoo D, Kim JW, Park SW, Shin JS and Cheon J. (2012). A magnetic switch for the control of cell death signalling in *in vitro* and *in vivo* systems. *Nature Mater.*, **11**:1038–1043.